The Genetic Plate

Exploring the World of Engineered Foods

Copyright Notice

Disclaimer

This book falls within the realm of nonfiction in the field of health. The information presented here is intended solely for general informational purposes and should not be considered a replacement for professional medical advice, diagnosis, or treatment. It is imperative to always seek guidance from a qualified healthcare provider or physician regarding any inquiries you may have about a medical condition. Please do not disregard professional medical advice or delay seeking it based on the content found in this book.

Contents

Introduction

In a world where the boundaries of science and technology continually expand, our plates have undergone a remarkable transformation. From the ancient rhythms of sowing and reaping to the precise choreography of genetic manipulation, the food we consume has evolved as a canvas for innovation and a reflection of our ever-changing relationship with the natural world.

"The Genetic Plate: Exploring the World of Engineered Foods" invites you on a captivating journey through the intersection of science, agriculture, and culinary artistry. This book is a window into the extraordinary story of genetically modified (GM) foods, a story that is reshaping the landscapes of our fields, the choices in our supermarkets, and the conversation at our dinner tables.

As we open this culinary adventure, we will explore the remarkable feats of science that have allowed us to tailor our crops to thrive in the face of adversity, from pests to droughts. We will delve into the quest for nutritional enhancement and the pursuit of a healthier, more sustainable food system. Along the way, we'll confront the intriguing questions of ethics, environmental impact, and the future of our global food supply.

But this book is not merely a chronicle of genetic engineering in agriculture; it is a celebration of the creative spirit that has shaped our food for millennia. It is an exploration of the curious and innovative minds that have sought to feed the world in the face of unprecedented challenges. "The Genetic Plate" is an ode to the ingenuity that has always defined our species and an examination of the potential and the perils that accompany it.

Let's, traverse the lush fields of GM crops, savor the fruits of the labors of pioneering scientists, and sample the debates, dilemmas, and dreams that compose the genetic plate before us. Welcome to a world where science and cuisine meet, where engineered foods are transforming the way we eat and think about what we eat.

Chapter 1

A Bite of Science

Genetic modification, often referred to as genetic engineering or biotechnology, is a powerful tool that has revolutionized agriculture and food production. It involves the deliberate manipulation of an organism's genetic material to introduce specific traits or characteristics. One of the key areas where genetic modification has had a significant impact is in altering the nutritional profile of foods.

Genetic modification in the context of food typically involves the introduction, deletion, or modification of genes in plants or animals. The goal is to confer specific traits or characteristics to these organisms, with a focus on enhancing their nutritional value, taste, or resistance to pests and environmental conditions.

Altering Nutritional Content

Enhancing nutrient levels in food through genetic modification is one of the significant objectives of biotechnology in agriculture. This approach aims to address nutritional deficiencies and improve the overall health and well-being of people around the world. Here are some key points to discuss the reasons for genetically modifying food to enhance nutrient levels:

1. **Alleviating Malnutrition:** Malnutrition, both undernutrition and overnutrition, is a pressing global issue. Genetically

modified (GM) crops can be designed to provide essential nutrients that are lacking in the diets of many people, particularly in developing countries. For instance, crops can be engineered to be rich in vitamins, minerals, and other nutrients, addressing deficiencies that can lead to health problems. Golden Rice is one of the most well-known examples of genetically modified food developed to enhance nutrient levels. It has been engineered to contain higher levels of provitamin A (beta-carotene), which the body converts into vitamin A. Vitamin A deficiency can lead to blindness and other health issues, particularly in areas where rice is a dietary staple.

2.   **Reducing Health-Related Costs:** By improving the nutrient content of staple crops, genetic modification can help reduce the prevalence of diet-related diseases. For example, increasing the levels of essential nutrients in crops may help lower the incidence of diet-related health issues such as anemia, night blindness, and immune system deficiencies. This can, in turn, reduce healthcare costs and improve overall public health.

3.   **Sustainable Nutrition:** Enhancing nutrient levels in food through genetic modification is part of a broader strategy for achieving sustainable nutrition. This approach can help reduce the reliance on

nutritional supplements and fortification programs, making it more accessible and cost-effective for populations in need.

4. **Environmental Considerations:** In some cases, enhancing nutrient levels in crops can lead to increased crop productivity and reduced agricultural waste. This is particularly relevant in regions where nutrient-poor soil is a challenge. By improving the nutrient content of crops, farmers may achieve better yields with fewer inputs.

Enhancing nutrient levels in food through genetic modification is a compelling reason to harness biotechnology to improve the quality of our food supply. By increasing the nutrient content of crops, we can combat malnutrition, reduce health-related costs, and work toward more sustainable and health-conscious agricultural practices.

The Science Behind Genetic Modification

Genetic modification, also known as genetic engineering or biotechnology, is a complex scientific process that involves the deliberate manipulation of an organism's genetic material, typically DNA. This technology has a wide range of applications in various fields, from agriculture to medicine. Let's delve into the key components of the science behind genetic modification:

Isolating Genetic Material

Isolating genetic material, typically DNA or RNA, is a fundamental step in various biological and molecular biology techniques, including DNA sequencing, PCR (Polymerase Chain Reaction), genetic engineering, and genetic testing. The process of isolating genetic material involves breaking down cellular structures and extracting the nucleic acids while preserving their integrity for further analysis. The process involves the following steps:

1. **Sample Collection:** The first step is to obtain a biological sample that contains the genetic material of interest. This can be anything from cells, tissues, blood, saliva, hair, or even environmental

samples like soil or water, depending on the research or diagnostic requirements.

2. **Cell Disruption:** In order to access the genetic material inside cells, the cell's integrity must be disrupted. This can be done using various methods, including:

- **Mechanical methods:** Homogenization, grinding, or mortar and pestle can physically break down cell walls.

- **Chemical methods:** Detergents like SDS (sodium dodecyl sulfate) can dissolve cell membranes.

- **Enzymatic methods:** Proteinase K can digest proteins that protect the genetic material.

3. **Centrifugation:** After cell disruption, a centrifuge is often used to separate the cellular debris, proteins, and other components from the genetic material. This results in a supernatant containing the nucleic acids.

4. **Precipitation:** To concentrate the nucleic acids further, ethanol or isopropanol can be added to the supernatant. This causes the nucleic acids to precipitate out of the solution.

5. **Purification:** The precipitated nucleic acids can contain impurities like proteins and other cellular contaminants. Purification methods, such as column chromatography or magnetic bead-based methods, are used to separate the

genetic material from these impurities.

6. **Washing:** Washing steps are performed to remove any remaining contaminants and ensure the purity of the genetic material.

7. **Elution:** The final step involves eluting the purified genetic material from the purification matrix or beads, resulting in a solution of isolated DNA or RNA.

It's important to note that the specific methods and protocols for isolating genetic material can vary depending on the source of the genetic material and the intended downstream applications. For example, the isolation of DNA from a blood sample differs from that of RNA from a plant leaf.

Isolated genetic material can then be used for various purposes, including genetic testing, gene sequencing, genetic engineering, forensic analysis, and more. The quality and purity of the isolated genetic material are critical, as any contaminants or degradation can affect the accuracy and reliability of subsequent analyses.

Target Gene Selection

In the context of genetically modified (GM) foods, target gene selection is a crucial step in the development of genetically engineered crops. The primary goal is to select and introduce specific genes into a crop's genome to impart desirable traits. Here are some key considerations and factors in target gene selection for GM food:

1.   **Desired Traits:** The most important consideration in target gene selection for GM foods is the desired trait or traits that the crop should possess. These traits can vary widely and may include resistance to pests, tolerance to herbicides, improved nutritional content, extended shelf life, or enhanced yield. The target genes should encode proteins or regulatory elements responsible for these traits.

2.   **Gene Silencing:** In some cases, target genes are chosen to facilitate gene silencing, which can lead to reduced expression of specific undesirable traits, such as browning in fruits or the synthesis

of anti-nutritional compounds.

3. **Crossbreeding Compatibility:** It's important to consider whether the introduced target gene will be compatible with traditional breeding methods, as this can impact the development of new crop varieties and the incorporation of the desired traits into a wider gene pool.

Once target genes are selected, the genetic modification process involves their insertion into the plant's genome, followed by extensive testing and evaluation to ensure that the GM crops meet safety, environmental, and performance standards. Target gene selection in GM food is a complex process that balances various scientific, regulatory, ethical, and consumer-related considerations to develop crops with improved traits.

Plasmid Vectors

Plasmid vectors play a significant role in the development of genetically modified (GM) foods. These small, circular pieces of DNA can carry specific genes of interest and are used to introduce desired traits into crops. Plasmid vectors are crucial tools in the genetic engineering of plants for various purposes, including pest resistance, herbicide tolerance, improved nutritional content, and more. Here's a discussion of the role of plasmid vectors in GM foods:

1.   **Gene Insertion:** Plasmid vectors are engineered to contain the target genes that encode the desired traits. These genes can be derived from various sources, including other plant species, bacteria, or even animals. The plasmid acts as a carrier to transport these genes into the target plant's genome.

2.   **Plant Transformation:** To create GM crops, the plasmid vectors are introduced into plant cells through a process called transformation. This can be achieved using different methods, such as Agrobacterium-mediated transformation or biolistic (gene gun) transformation. The plasmid vectors deliver the target genes into the plant's DNA.

Plasmid vectors can be designed to carry multiple genes, allowing the development of GM crops with multiple desirable traits. For instance, a single plasmid vector might carry genes for both pest resistance and herbicide tolerance.

Plasmid vectors may also contain marker genes, which are not the primary genes of interest but serve as indicators of successful transformation. These marker genes can help in selecting and identifying transformed cells or plants.

In summary, plasmid vectors are essential tools in the genetic modification of crops for GM foods. They enable the precise introduction of target genes into the plant genome, leading to the expression of desired traits. However, their use is subject to rigorous scientific, regulatory, and ethical considerations to ensure the safety and acceptability of GM foods in the market.

Restriction Enzymes

Restriction enzymes (also known as restriction endonucleases) are essential tools in genetic engineering and the development of genetically modified (GM) foods. These enzymes recognize specific DNA sequences, known as recognition sites, and cleave the DNA at those sites. They are categorized into different types based on their properties and functions, and they serve various purposes in GM food development.

Types of Restriction Enzymes:

1. **Type I Restriction Enzymes:** Type I enzymes recognize a specific DNA sequence, but they cleave the DNA at some distance from the recognition site. They are multifunctional enzymes with separate recognition, cleavage, and DNA modification domains.

2. **Type II Restriction Enzymes:** Type II enzymes are the most commonly used in genetic engineering. They recognize specific palindromic DNA sequences, cleave the DNA at or near the recognition site, and are easy to manipulate. Examples of Type II restriction enzymes include EcoRI, HindIII, and BamHI.

3.   **Type III Restriction Enzymes:** Type III enzymes, like Type I enzymes, cleave DNA at some distance from the recognition site. They also possess DNA modification activity. These enzymes are less commonly used in genetic engineering.

4.   **Type IV Restriction Enzymes:** Type IV enzymes recognize and modify DNA, but they do not cleave it. They have specific roles in DNA methylation and protection against foreign DNA.

Uses of Restriction Enzymes in GM Foods:

1. **Gene Cloning:** Restriction enzymes are used to cut both the target gene and the plasmid vector at specific recognition sites. This allows for the creation of complementary ends on the DNA

fragments, making it possible to ligate the target gene into the vector. The modified plasmid can then be introduced into the host organism to express the desired trait.

2. **Creation of Recombinant DNA:** Restriction enzymes are employed to cut the DNA of interest and generate fragments with compatible ends. When combined with the plasmid vector, these fragments create recombinant DNA molecules. This recombinant DNA carries the target gene and is a fundamental step in GM crop development.

3. **Stacking Traits:** In the development of GM crops with multiple desirable traits, different target genes can be introduced

into the same plasmid vector. This is made possible by using compatible restriction enzyme recognition sites in the vector and the target genes. This enables the creation of crops with multiple beneficial characteristics.

4. **Gene Silencing:** In some cases, restriction enzymes are used to create constructs for gene silencing, such as RNA interference (RNAi). These constructs are designed to suppress the expression of specific genes in GM crops, which can be used to control undesirable traits.

Restriction enzymes, particularly Type II restriction enzymes, are fundamental tools in the development of GM foods. They enable the precise manipulation of DNA to introduce and control target genes, allowing for the creation of crops with enhanced characteristics and traits. The use of restriction enzymes in GM food development is subject to rigorous regulatory scrutiny to ensure safety for both human consumption and the environment.

Ligases

DNA ligases are responsible for joining or ligating DNA fragments together, sealing nicks or gaps in the DNA molecule. This process is crucial for creating recombinant DNA molecules, including those used in GM crop development. DNA ligases used in genetic engineering are generally of two main types: DNA ligase I and DNA ligase IV.

1. DNA Ligase I:

- **Type I DNA Ligases:** These enzymes are typically involved in DNA replication and repair in living organisms. They seal nicks in the phosphodiester backbone of DNA, helping to ensure the continuity of the DNA strands. Type I DNA ligases are less commonly used in genetic engineering for creating GM crops and are not typically found as a specific tool for that purpose.

2. DNA Ligase IV:

- **Type II DNA Ligases (including DNA Ligase IV):** In genetic engineering and biotechnology, Type II DNA ligases, especially DNA Ligase IV, are commonly used to ligate DNA fragments together.

DNA Ligase IV is particularly important for the development of GM foods.

Uses of DNA Ligases in GM Food Production:

1. **Gene Cloning:** DNA ligases play a crucial role in gene cloning, which is the process of making multiple copies of a specific DNA fragment. After DNA fragments are cut using restriction enzymes, DNA ligases are used to join these fragments into plasmid vectors. This process allows for the creation of recombinant DNA molecules containing the target genes. These recombinant DNA molecules can then be introduced into host organisms (e.g., crop plants) for gene expression.

2. **Recombinant DNA Construct Formation:**
   In GM food development, DNA ligases are
   used to create recombinant DNA
   constructs containing the desired traits.
   DNA fragments, such as regulatory
   elements, promoters, target genes, and
   marker genes, are ligated together to
   form these constructs. The constructs are
   designed to control the expression of the
   target gene and can be introduced into
   the host organism for expression.

3. **Transformation:** After the formation of
   recombinant DNA constructs, DNA ligases
   ensure the integrity of these constructs
   before they are introduced into the host
   organism (usually a plant in GM crop
   development). DNA ligases help maintain

the structural integrity of the recombinant DNA, ensuring the successful expression of the introduced genes.

4. **Transgene Stabilization:** DNA ligases are essential for the stable integration of transgenes (the introduced genes) into the host organism's genome. This ensures that the transgenes are maintained and expressed in subsequent generations of GM crops.

5. **Marker Gene Insertion:** In some cases, marker genes are used in GM crops to indicate successful gene insertion. DNA ligases are involved in ligating these marker genes with the target genes into plasmid vectors, allowing for the

selection of transformed plants.

6. **Gene Silencing Constructs:** DNA ligases are used in creating constructs for gene silencing, such as RNA interference (RNAi). These constructs are designed to suppress the expression of specific genes in GM crops, which can be used to control undesirable traits.

DNA ligases, particularly Type II DNA ligases, are essential enzymes in the development of GM foods. They are used to join DNA fragments, create recombinant DNA constructs, and ensure the stable integration of transgenes into the host organism's genome. This enables the development of GM crops with enhanced characteristics and traits. The use of DNA ligases in GM food production is subject to rigorous regulatory scrutiny to ensure the safety and environmental compatibility of the modified crops.

Selection and Expression

Selection and expression are crucial steps in the production of genetically modified (GM) foods, particularly GM crops. These steps are vital for ensuring that the introduced genes are effectively incorporated into the host organism's genome and that they produce the desired traits or characteristics. Here's a discussion of selection and expression in GM food production:

1. Selection:

a. Tissue Culture and Regeneration: After the introduction of foreign genes into the host organism, the transformed cells are typically placed in tissue culture. This step allows the cells to multiply and regenerate, eventually forming whole plants. The selection process begins at this stage to identify cells that have successfully integrated the transgenes.

b. Marker Genes: To identify transformed cells, marker genes are often included in the genetic construct along with the target genes. These marker genes can confer specific traits, such as resistance to antibiotics or the ability to produce a specific pigment, which makes it easier to identify and select the transformed cells. Cells that express the marker gene are presumed to carry the target gene as well.

c. Antibiotic Resistance: In many cases, antibiotic resistance genes are used as selectable markers. Transformed cells containing the antibiotic resistance gene can survive in the presence of antibiotics, while untransformed cells cannot. This allows for the selection of transformed cells during tissue culture.

d. Molecular Analysis: In addition to marker genes, molecular techniques, such as polymerase chain reaction (PCR) and DNA analysis, are used to confirm the presence of the target genes. These techniques ensure that the desired genes have been successfully integrated into the host organism's genome.

2. Expression:

a. Verification of Gene Expression: Once transgenic plants have been generated, it's essential to confirm that the target genes are actively expressing the desired traits. This involves monitoring the plants for the production of specific proteins or other characteristics associated with the introduced genes.

b. Regulatory Elements: In GM food production, the expression of the target genes is controlled by regulatory elements, including promoters, enhancers, and terminators. These elements determine when and where the genes are active in the plant. For example, a promoter can dictate that a pest-resistant gene is only expressed when the plant is attacked by pests.

c. Environmental Factors: Environmental conditions, such as light, temperature, and nutrient availability, can influence the expression of target genes. Researchers and growers must understand how the expression of these genes is affected by environmental factors to optimize the desired traits in GM crops.

d. Stability of Gene Expression: Ensuring the stability of gene expression across generations of GM crops is important. The introduced genes should continue to produce the desired traits consistently, and this stability is assessed in field trials and during regulatory evaluations.

e. Monitoring of Off-Target Effects: In GM food production, it's essential to monitor for unintended or off-target effects of gene expression. This includes assessing potential impacts on non-target organisms, ecosystems, and human health.

f. Field Trials and Evaluation: Before GM crops are approved for commercial cultivation, they typically undergo field trials to assess their performance, safety, and environmental impact. Field trials provide an opportunity to evaluate the expression of target genes under real-world conditions.

g. Regulatory Approval: The release of GM foods into the market is subject to regulatory scrutiny in many countries. Regulatory agencies assess the safety of GM crops for human consumption and the environment, as well as their compliance with labeling and traceability requirements. Selection and expression are critical steps in GM food production, ensuring that the introduced genes are successfully integrated into the host organism's genome and that they produce the desired traits. These steps involve the use of selectable markers, regulatory elements for gene control, environmental considerations, stability assessments, monitoring for off-target effects, and regulatory evaluations. The resulting GM crops are developed to address various agricultural and food production challenges, such as pest resistance, herbicide tolerance, improved nutritional content, and increased yield.

Characterization and Evaluation

Characterization and evaluation play vital roles in the production of genetically modified (GM) foods. These steps involve comprehensive testing and analysis to ensure the safety, efficacy, and regulatory compliance of GM crops. Here's a discussion of characterization and evaluation in GM food production:

Characterization

1. **Molecular Characterization:** This step involves the detailed analysis of the GM plant's molecular profile. It includes the

identification and verification of the introduced genes, their structure, and their location within the plant's genome.

2.   **Gene Expression Analysis:** Molecular characterization includes assessing the expression of the introduced genes. It ensures that the target genes are actively producing the desired proteins and traits.

3.   **Stability Assessment:** The stability of gene expression across generations is evaluated to confirm that the introduced genes continue to function as expected in subsequent generations of the GM crop.

4.   **Assessment of Off-Target Effects:** Researchers assess potential unintended or off-target effects of genetic modification. This involves identifying any

unexpected changes in the plant's physiology, biochemistry, or molecular profile.

5. **Allergenicity Testing:** Characterization includes allergenicity assessments to determine whether the GM crop's introduced proteins have the potential to induce allergic reactions in humans.

6. **Toxicity Testing:** To ensure the safety of GM foods, toxicity studies are conducted to assess whether consuming the GM crop poses any health risks. These tests are usually performed on animals.

7. **Environmental Impact Assessment:** Researchers evaluate the potential environmental impact of the GM crop, including its effects on non-target

organisms, soil quality, and ecosystems.

Evaluation

1. **Field Trials:** GM crops undergo field trials to assess their performance under real-world conditions. These trials help determine how the GM crop behaves in terms of growth, yield, resistance to pests and diseases, and adaptability to local environments.

2. **Environmental Risk Assessment:** Evaluations are made regarding the potential environmental risks associated with the cultivation of GM crops. This includes assessing the likelihood of gene flow to wild relatives and the development of herbicide-resistant

weeds.

3. **Comparative Analysis:** GM crops are compared to their non-GM counterparts to assess the effectiveness of the introduced traits. This includes evaluating factors such as crop yield, nutritional content, and resistance to pests or diseases.

4. **Allergenicity and Toxicity Testing:** Comprehensive allergenicity and toxicity testing is conducted to ensure the safety of GM foods. This involves animal studies to evaluate potential health risks and allergenic reactions.

5. **Nutritional Assessment:** The nutritional content of GM crops is compared to that of non-GM counterparts to confirm that

the introduced traits do not negatively affect nutritional value.

6. **Human Health Assessment:** Assessments are made to determine whether the consumption of GM crops has any impact on human health. This may include clinical studies and monitoring of populations that regularly consume GM foods.

7. **Regulatory Approval:** The release of GM foods into the market is subject to regulatory scrutiny in many countries. Regulatory agencies evaluate the safety, environmental impact, and compliance with labeling and traceability requirements.

8. **Public Acceptance:** Evaluating public attitudes and acceptance of GM foods is

crucial, as consumer perceptions can influence marketability. Public engagement and education efforts may be conducted to address concerns and promote transparency.

Characterization and evaluation in GM food production are extensive processes designed to ensure the safety, efficacy, and regulatory compliance of GM crops. These steps involve a combination of molecular analyses, field trials, environmental risk assessments, safety testing, nutritional assessments, and regulatory evaluations. The aim is to provide consumers with GM foods that are safe, sustainable, and beneficial while addressing various agricultural and food production challenges.

Regulation and Safety Assessment

Before genetically modified organisms are released into the environment or introduced into the food supply, they typically undergo rigorous safety assessments and regulatory scrutiny. These assessments evaluate the potential risks and benefits of the modified organism.

Commercialization

Once a genetically modified organism is deemed safe and effective, it can be commercialized. This may involve obtaining regulatory approvals, patenting the technology, and scaling up production.

Continuous Monitoring

After commercialization, the genetically modified organisms are often subject to ongoing monitoring for safety and environmental impact. This includes post-market surveillance to ensure the technology's long-term safety.

It's important to note that genetic modification is a precise and controlled process, but it also raises various ethical, environmental, and regulatory considerations. The science behind genetic modification continues to evolve, and emerging technologies like CRISPR-Cas9 have made genetic editing more precise and accessible. Understanding the science behind genetic modification is crucial for

informed discussions and decision-making
regarding its applications and implications.

Chapter 2

Genes used in genetically modified (GM) foods, also known as genetically modified organisms (GMOs), are sourced from a variety of organisms, often with the aim of introducing specific desirable traits into crops. These genes can come from different organisms, including bacteria, plants, and even virus. Here are the key sources of genes used in GM foods:

Bacteria

Bacteria are a common and important source of genes used in genetically modified (GM) foods. Bacterial genes play a crucial role in the development of GM crops, particularly in conferring resistance to pests, diseases, and herbicides. Here is a detailed discussion of bacteria as a source of genes for GM foods:

1. Bt Genes (Bacillus thuringiensis):

- One of the most widely used sources of bacterial genes in GM foods is Bacillus thuringiensis (Bt). Bt is a naturally occurring soil bacterium that produces insecticidal proteins. These Bt proteins, when incorporated into GM crops, can provide built-in protection against specific insect pests.

- The Bt genes produce toxins that target the digestive systems of certain insects, making them an effective and environmentally friendly alternative to chemical pesticides.

- GM crops containing Bt genes are engineered to express these proteins, making the plant resistant to insect damage. Common Bt crops include Bt cotton, Bt corn, and Bt potatoes.

2. Agrobacterium tumefaciens:

- Agrobacterium tumefaciens is a soil bacterium that has been used in GM crop development. It has a natural ability to transfer genetic material into plant cells. Scientists have harnessed this capability to introduce specific genes into plant genomes.

- Agrobacterium-mediated genetic transformation has been crucial in the development of various GM crops, including soybeans, cotton, and several vegetables.

3. Nitrogen-Fixing Bacteria:

- Some GM crops, like certain varieties of soybeans and alfalfa, have been engineered to improve their nitrogen-fixing capabilities. This is achieved by introducing genes from nitrogen-fixing bacteria, such as Bradyrhizobium japonicum. These genes enable the plants to form a symbiotic relationship with these bacteria, enhancing their ability to capture nitrogen from the atmosphere and convert it into a form that can be used for plant growth.

4. Antibiotic Resistance Marker Genes:

- In the early stages of GM crop development, antibiotic resistance genes from bacteria were sometimes used as selectable markers during the genetic modification process. These genes helped scientists identify and select successfully transformed plant cells. However, the use of antibiotic resistance genes has raised concerns about the potential transfer of antibiotic resistance to other organisms. As a result, there has been a move toward using alternative selection markers.

Plants

Plants serve as a significant source of genes used in the development of genetically modified (GM) foods. These genes are selected and introduced into target crops to confer various desirable traits, such as resistance to pests, tolerance to herbicides, improved nutritional content, and enhanced adaptation to environmental conditions. Here's a discussion of plants as a source of genes for GM foods:

1. Pest Resistance Genes:

- Many GM crops are engineered with genes from other plants to provide resistance against insect pests. For example, the Bt (Bacillus thuringiensis) gene, which produces insecticidal proteins, has been used extensively in GM crops like Bt cotton and Bt corn.

2. Herbicide Tolerance Genes:

- Some GM crops are designed to withstand specific herbicides. Genes that confer herbicide tolerance are introduced to enhance a crop's ability to survive herbicide applications. Commonly used genes include the EPSPS (5-enolpyruvylshikimate-3-phosphate synthase) gene, which provides tolerance to glyphosate (Roundup), and the ALS (acetolactate synthase) gene, which confers tolerance to certain herbicides.

3. Disease Resistance Genes:

- Genes from other plants or relatives of the target crop may be incorporated to enhance disease resistance. For instance, resistance genes from wild tomato species have been used to improve the resistance of cultivated tomato plants to diseases like late blight.

4. Environmental Stress Tolerance Genes:

- To help crops withstand environmental stresses, such as drought, salinity, or extreme temperatures, genes from other plant species or related varieties are introduced. These genes can enhance the crop's resilience and adaptation to challenging conditions.

5. Nutritional Enhancement Genes:

- Some GM crops are developed to be nutritionally enhanced. Genes from other plants can be utilized to increase the content of specific nutrients. An example is "Golden Rice," which contains genes from maize and a soil bacterium to boost pro-vitamin A (beta-carotene) levels.

6. Delayed Ripening Genes:

- Genes responsible for delaying the ripening of fruits have been employed to extend the shelf life of certain GM fruits and vegetables, reducing food waste during transportation and storage.

7. Non-Browning Genes:

- Certain GM crops have been designed to resist browning upon injury or exposure to air. Genes from other plants can be used to inhibit the enzymatic processes responsible for browning, as seen in GM apples and potatoes.

8. Resistance to Abiotic Stress:

- Genes from other plants may be introduced to confer resistance to abiotic stress factors like high salinity, heavy metals, or toxic substances in the soil, making crops more adaptable to challenging growing conditions.

9. Wild Relatives and Closely Related Species:

- The genetic diversity present in wild relatives or closely related species of cultivated crops is a valuable source of genes for GM crop development. These genes can introduce novel traits and enhance the genetic diversity of commercial crops.

Viral Genes

Viral genes have been used as a source of genes in the development of genetically modified (GM) foods, particularly in the field of crop biotechnology. Viral genes are often employed to enhance the resistance of crops to specific diseases or to improve the overall health and yield of plants. Here's a discussion of the use of viral genes in GM foods:

1. Virus Resistance:

- One of the primary applications of viral genes in GM foods is to confer resistance to viral diseases that can devastate crop yields. Plants are often vulnerable to a variety of plant viruses that can lead to stunted growth, reduced crop quality, and yield losses.

- To enhance viral resistance, specific viral genes or gene fragments are introduced into the genome of the target crop. These genes produce viral coat proteins or other components that, when expressed in the plant, trigger a defense response against the virus.

2. Papaya Ringspot Virus-Resistant Papaya:

- A well-known example of GM food developed with viral genes is the "Rainbow" papaya. This genetically modified papaya was engineered to resist the destructive Papaya Ringspot Virus (PRSV).

- In this case, a gene from the PRSV was used to create a coat protein that, when expressed in the papaya plant, protected it from infection by the virus. This GM papaya variety helped save the Hawaiian papaya industry, which was under severe threat from PRSV.

3. Tomato Yellow Leaf Curl Virus-Resistant Tomatoes:

- GM tomatoes have been developed with viral genes to enhance resistance to the Tomato Yellow Leaf Curl Virus (TYLCV). Genes from the TYLCV, along with other viral components, have been used to create GM tomatoes that are less susceptible to this destructive virus.

4. Non-Viral Diseases:

- While viral genes are primarily used for virus resistance, some GM crops may incorporate genes that help protect against non-viral diseases. These genes may include sequences related to fungal or bacterial pathogens that can impact plant health.

- In some cases, these genes function by stimulating the plant's natural defense mechanisms to combat pathogens.

Synthetic Genes:

Synthetic genes have been used in genetically modified (GM) foods to introduce specific traits or characteristics into crops. Here are some examples of the application of synthetic genes in GM foods:

1.   **Bt Cotton:**

- One of the most well-known applications of synthetic genes in GM crops is in Bt cotton. Synthetic genes derived from the bacterium Bacillus thuringiensis were incorporated into cotton plants. These genes produce a protein toxic to certain insect pests, such as the cotton bollworm. This genetic modification has significantly reduced the need for chemical insecticides in cotton farming, leading to increased yields and reduced environmental impact.

2.   **Golden Rice:**

- Golden Rice is a genetically modified variety of rice designed to combat vitamin A deficiency, a major health issue in many developing countries. Synthetic genes were used to introduce beta-carotene biosynthesis pathways into rice plants, giving the rice grains a yellowish color. Beta-carotene is a precursor of vitamin A, and this modification aimed to increase the nutritional value of rice, particularly for populations relying heavily on rice as a staple food.

3. **Drought-Tolerant Crops:**

- Synthetic genes have been utilized in GM crops to improve drought tolerance. By introducing genes that enhance water-use efficiency and reduce water stress, crops like maize and soybeans have been developed to thrive under limited water conditions. This has the potential to increase crop yields in regions prone to drought.

4. **Herbicide-Tolerant Crops:**

- Certain GM crops have been engineered with synthetic genes to be tolerant to specific herbicides. For example, glyphosate-tolerant crops like Roundup Ready soybeans and maize have been modified to withstand glyphosate-based herbicides, simplifying weed control in agricultural fields.

5. **Delayed Ripening Tomatoes:**

- Synthetic genes have been used to develop tomatoes with delayed ripening. This modification extends the shelf life of tomatoes and reduces post-harvest losses. It also allows for tomatoes to be harvested at their peak ripeness before they become too soft for transportation and consumption.

6. **Fruit and Vegetable Quality Enhancement:**

- Synthetic genes have been employed to improve the quality of fruits and vegetables. For instance, the Arctic Apple is a genetically modified apple that has been engineered to resist browning when sliced, which can reduce food waste and improve the consumer experience.

These examples showcase the diverse applications of synthetic genes in GM foods, addressing issues related to pest resistance, nutritional content, environmental impact, and food quality. However, it's important to note that the adoption and acceptance of GM foods vary across regions and are influenced by factors such as regulatory policies, public perception, and the ability to demonstrate safety and benefits. Rigorous safety assessments are typically conducted to ensure that these genetic modifications do not pose risks to human health or the environment.

The selection of genes and their sources is determined by the specific goals of GM crop development, which may include improving crop yield, enhancing nutritional content, reducing the need for chemical pesticides, or conferring resistance to environmental factors. Regulatory agencies assess the safety of these GM crops before they are approved for commercial cultivation and consumption. Additionally, labeling and traceability requirements ensure that consumers are informed about the presence of GM ingredients in their food.

Chapter 3

The Frankenfood Controversy

Genetically engineered foods, often referred to as "GMOs" (genetically modified organisms), have been a subject of intense controversy and debate for decades. On one hand, proponents argue that GMOs hold the potential to address food security challenges, reduce pesticide use, and improve crop yields. On the other hand, critics express concerns about the long-term health and environmental consequences, corporate control over agriculture, and ethical considerations.

Benefits of Genetically Engineered Foods

Genetically engineered foods, often referred to as genetically modified (GM) or genetically modified organisms (GMOs), offer several potential benefits in agriculture and the food industry. While the adoption and acceptance of GM foods vary worldwide, the technology behind them has the potential to address various challenges. Here are some of the key benefits associated with genetically engineered foods:

1. **Increased Crop Yields:** GM crops are often designed to resist pests, diseases, or environmental stressors, which results in higher crop yields. Enhanced resistance

to insects and diseases reduces crop losses, ensuring that more food reaches the market and can contribute to global food security.

2. **Reduced Pesticide Use:** Pest-resistant GM crops, such as Bt cotton and Bt corn, produce a protein toxic to specific insect pests. Farmers growing these crops often use fewer chemical pesticides, reducing potential harm to the environment and decreasing the need for costly pesticide applications.

3. **Improved Crop Tolerance to Environmental Conditions:** Some GM crops are engineered to withstand adverse environmental conditions like drought, extreme temperatures, or soil

salinity. This resilience helps crops thrive in regions where these conditions are common and can lead to more reliable harvests.

4.   **Enhanced Nutritional Content:** Genetic engineering can be used to enrich the nutritional content of crops. For instance, Golden Rice has been developed to contain higher levels of provitamin A (beta-carotene), addressing vitamin A deficiency in regions where rice is a dietary staple.

5.   **Extended Shelf Life:** Genetic modification can enhance the shelf life of fruits and vegetables by delaying ripening or reducing susceptibility to spoilage. This can reduce food waste and increase the

availability of fresh produce.

6. **Reduced Post-Harvest Losses:** Crops can be engineered to be less susceptible to bruising, damage, or spoilage during transportation and storage. This is particularly beneficial in regions with inadequate infrastructure for food preservation and transportation.

7. **Improved Quality and Flavor:** Genetic modification can lead to the production of fruits and vegetables with better taste, texture, and appearance. This can increase consumer acceptance and consumption of these foods.

8. **Lower Production Costs:** GM crops that require fewer pesticide applications, less water, and reduced soil tilling can

result in lower production costs for farmers. This can contribute to more economically sustainable agriculture.

9. **Disease Resistance in Livestock:** In addition to crops, genetic engineering can be applied to livestock. For example, GM animals can be engineered to be resistant to specific diseases. This can enhance animal welfare and reduce the need for antibiotics in animal agriculture.

10. **Sustainability and Reduced Environmental Impact:** By reducing the need for chemical pesticides and fertilizers, GM crops can contribute to more environmentally sustainable farming practices. This, in turn, can help conserve biodiversity and reduce the

environmental impact of agriculture.

11.   **Meeting Global Food Demand:** As the global population continues to grow, genetically engineered foods have the potential to help meet the increasing demand for food by improving crop productivity and sustainability.

Concerns Surrounding Genetically Engineered Foods

Genetically engineered foods have generated a range of concerns and controversies. While these foods offer potential benefits, such as increased crop yields and reduced pesticide use, there are several key concerns associated with their development, commercialization, and consumption. Here are the primary concerns surrounding genetically engineered foods:

1. **Environmental Concerns:**

a. **Ecological Impact:** GM crops can crossbreed with wild relatives, potentially creating hybrid plants that may affect ecosystems. This genetic flow can lead to unintended environmental consequences.

b. **Emergence of Resistant Pests and Weeds:** Continuous cultivation of pest-resistant GM crops may lead to the development of resistance in targeted pests. Similarly, herbicide-resistant crops can contribute to the emergence of herbicide-resistant weeds, potentially leading to more chemical use.

c. **Biodiversity Loss:** The widespread adoption of GM monocultures may reduce genetic diversity within a crop species. This can make crops more susceptible to diseases and pests, endangering food security.

2. **Human Health Concerns:**

a. **Allergenicity:** Genetic modification can introduce new proteins into foods, which may trigger allergies in some individuals. Proper allergenicity testing is crucial to ensure the safety of GM foods.

b. **Unintended Effects:** The genetic modification process can have unintended and unpredictable effects on the composition of the modified plant. These unintended effects need to be thoroughly assessed for potential health risks.

c. **Long-Term Health Implications:** There is ongoing debate about the potential long-term health effects of consuming GM foods, as well as the need for extensive, independent, long-term studies.

3.   **Ethical and Social Concerns:**

a. **Ownership and Intellectual Property Rights:** The patenting of GM seeds by biotechnology companies raises concerns about control over the food supply and the influence of corporate interests on agriculture. It can also limit access to GM technology for small farmers in developing countries.

b. **Consumer Choice and Labeling:** Many people want to know whether the foods they consume contain GM ingredients. Labeling of GM foods is a contentious issue, with some advocating for clear and transparent labeling, while others argue that it can stigmatize GM products.

4.   **Regulatory Oversight:**

a. **Regulatory Effectiveness:** Concerns have been raised about the adequacy and transparency of regulatory oversight for GM crops and foods. Some critics argue that the regulatory processes may not adequately address long-term safety concerns.

b. **Lack of Independent Research:** Some argue that the limited number of independent studies on GM crops and their safety is a concern. Independent research can help provide a more comprehensive understanding of potential risks.

5.   **Economic Concerns:**

a. **Market Control:** The consolidation of seed and chemical companies in the GM industry can lead to market monopolies and limit the choices available to farmers. Smaller and more diverse seed companies may struggle to compete.

b. **Economic Disparities:** In some cases, GM technology has led to economic disparities between large commercial farms that can afford GM seeds and smaller, resource-limited farms that cannot. The technology can potentially exacerbate social and economic inequality.

6. **Trade and Export Issues:**

a. **Export Constraints:** Some countries restrict or ban the import of GM crops and foods. This can create trade disputes and challenges for countries that grow GM crops.

b. **Segregation and Identity Preservation:** Ensuring the purity of non-GM crops in areas where GM crops are grown can be challenging. The coexistence of GM and non-GM crops is a significant concern for farmers.

7. **Unintended Crossbreeding:**

a. **Gene Flow:** GM crops can crossbreed with non-GM crops, leading to the unintentional presence of GM traits in non-GM crops. This can create difficulties in maintaining the purity of non-GM varieties.

Addressing these concerns and striking a balance between the potential benefits and risks of genetically engineered foods is a complex task. It involves rigorous scientific research, transparent regulatory processes, ethical considerations, and public engagement to ensure the responsible development and use of GM technology in agriculture and the food industry.

Regulatory Oversight

Regulatory oversight of genetically modified (GM) foods is essential to ensure their safety, proper labeling, and responsible development and commercialization. The regulatory landscape varies from country to country, but it generally involves a combination of government agencies, safety assessments, and labeling requirements. Here are the key aspects of regulatory oversight of GM foods:

1. **Regulatory Authorities:** Most countries have established regulatory bodies or agencies responsible for overseeing GM foods. In the United States, for example, the primary agency is the U.S. Food and Drug Administration (FDA), which collaborates with the U.S. Department of Agriculture (USDA) and the Environmental Protection Agency (EPA). In the European Union (EU), the European Food Safety Authority (EFSA) plays a central role.

2.   **Pre-Market Safety Assessments:** Before a GM food can be commercially cultivated or sold, it must undergo rigorous safety assessments. These assessments evaluate the potential risks to human health and the environment. Key aspects include:

a. **Environmental Risk Assessment:** This evaluates the potential ecological impact of GM crops, including their potential to crossbreed with wild relatives and their impact on non-target organisms.

b. **Food Safety Assessment:** This assesses the safety of GM foods for human consumption. It involves evaluating the introduced gene's function, potential allergenicity, and other factors that may affect food safety.

c. **Comparative Assessment:** This involves comparing the GM crop with its non-GM counterpart to identify any unintended changes in composition or quality.

3. **Transparency and Data Accessibility:** Regulatory oversight requires transparency in the submission of data and research findings by the developers of GM crops. Independent experts and regulatory agencies should have access to this data to conduct comprehensive safety assessments.

4. **Public Consultation:** In many countries, public consultation and input are integral to the regulatory process. The public is often invited to comment on proposed

GM crop approvals or undergo public hearings, allowing for a diversity of perspectives to be considered.

5. **Labeling Requirements:** GM foods may be subject to specific labeling requirements. Labeling informs consumers about the presence of GM ingredients in the products they purchase. Labeling may also extend to processed foods containing GM components or ingredients.

6. **Post-Market Surveillance:** Regulatory authorities often require ongoing monitoring and surveillance of GM crops and GM foods once they are on the market. This surveillance helps to detect and address any unforeseen issues or

unintended effects.

7.   **Coexistence and Identity Preservation:** To accommodate both GM and non-GM agriculture, regulatory frameworks may establish guidelines for coexistence and identity preservation. These measures aim to prevent unintended mixing of GM and non-GM crops and ensure that consumers have access to non-GM products if desired.

8.   **International Agreements:** Many countries adhere to international agreements and conventions related to GM foods. The Cartagena Protocol on Biosafety, for example, is an international treaty that regulates the international trade of GM organisms and aims to

protect biological diversity.

9. **Trade Considerations:** The regulation of GM foods can have implications for international trade. Trade partners may have different regulatory requirements, and trade disputes can arise when exporting GM crops or foods to countries with restrictive policies.

10. **Emerging Technologies:** As new genetic engineering techniques, such as CRISPR-Cas9, have emerged, regulatory agencies are adapting to address the regulatory challenges posed by these technologies.

11. **Adaptive Regulations:** Regulatory oversight is a dynamic process that should adapt to emerging scientific

knowledge and technological advancements. This adaptability ensures that regulatory frameworks remain robust and responsive to evolving circumstances.

The effectiveness of regulatory oversight depends on several factors, including the scientific rigor of safety assessments, the transparency of the regulatory process, public engagement, and the capacity of regulatory agencies to carry out their responsibilities. Striking a balance between ensuring safety and fostering innovation in biotechnology is an ongoing challenge, and regulatory frameworks continue to evolve to meet these challenges while addressing public concerns and expectations.

Consumer Awareness and Labeling

Consumer awareness and labeling of genetically modified (GM) foods are critical aspects of regulatory and ethical considerations in the food industry. These practices empower consumers to make informed choices about the products they purchase and consume. Let's discuss the significance of consumer awareness and labeling of GM foods:

1. **Informed Consumer Choice:** Labeling of GM foods provides consumers with information about the presence of genetically modified ingredients in products. This transparency allows individuals to make choices that align with their personal preferences, values,

or dietary needs.

2. **Allergen and Dietary Considerations:** Some individuals have specific dietary requirements or allergies. GM labeling helps these consumers avoid foods that may contain allergenic or otherwise problematic genetic modifications.

3. **Religious and Ethical Concerns:** Certain religious or ethical beliefs may prohibit the consumption of GM foods. Labeling allows consumers to adhere to their beliefs by making conscious food choices.

4. **Health and Environmental Concerns:** Some consumers are concerned about the potential health and environmental implications of GM foods. Clear labeling enables them to select products that

align with their values and concerns.

5. **Accurate Information:** Labeling ensures that information about GM content is accurate. It helps prevent misinformation and the spread of false or misleading claims about the presence or absence of GM ingredients.

6. **Public Trust and Confidence:** Transparent labeling fosters trust between consumers and food producers. It assures consumers that companies are providing accurate information about the products they offer.

7. **Public Engagement:** Labeling GM foods often involves public consultation and input. Engaging the public in the decision-making process regarding GM

labeling can help address a diverse range of perspectives and concerns.

8. **Global Trade and Harmonization:** Standardized GM labeling practices can facilitate international trade by ensuring that products conform to labeling requirements in different countries. This helps prevent trade disruptions and disputes.

9. **Monitoring and Traceability:** Labeling is a key component of traceability, which is crucial for tracking and managing GM products throughout the supply chain. In the event of a safety concern, traceability allows for more efficient recalls or investigations.

10. **Market Differentiation:** GM labeling can serve as a marketing tool for companies producing non-GM or organic products. Consumers who actively seek non-GM options can identify and support such products.

Despite these benefits, there are challenges and complexities associated with GM food labeling:

1. **Labeling Thresholds:** Determining the threshold at which a product should be labeled as containing GM ingredients can be challenging, particularly when it comes to adventitious presence (i.e., unintended trace amounts of GM material).

2. **Enforcement and Compliance:** Effective enforcement of labeling regulations is

essential to ensure that companies accurately label their products. Violations can be an issue, especially when companies attempt to conceal the presence of GM ingredients.

3. **Consumer Education:** For labeling to be meaningful, consumers need to be educated about what GM labeling means, the reasons behind it, and how to interpret labeling information.

4. **Global Variability:** Labeling regulations vary by country, leading to challenges in harmonizing global trade. Companies often need to navigate a complex patchwork of labeling requirements.

5. **Cost Implications:** There may be additional costs associated with labeling,

such as testing, record-keeping, and label design. Smaller producers may find compliance more burdensome.

6. **Resistance to GM Labeling:** In some cases, industry stakeholders or policymakers resist mandatory GM labeling, citing concerns about cost, complexity, or potential stigmatization of GM products.

7. **Consumer Acceptance:** Consumer acceptance of GM labeling can vary. Some consumers may embrace it as a matter of choice, while others may be indifferent or find it stigmatizing.

Consumer awareness and labeling of GM foods play a vital role in ensuring transparency, choice, and trust in the food supply chain. While there are challenges associated with GM labeling, it remains an important tool for empowering consumers to make informed decisions about the foods they purchase and consume. Effective, standardized, and transparent labeling practices contribute to a more informed and conscientious food industry.

The "Frankenfood" controversy is a complex and multifaceted debate, with both valid concerns and potential benefits. Genetic engineering has the potential to address critical agricultural and nutritional challenges, but it also raises questions about its long-term consequences for health, the environment, and societal well-being. Striking a balance between responsible innovation and safety is essential to navigate this controversial terrain and ensure that genetically engineered foods serve the interests of both producers and consumers.

Chapter 4

GM Crops Around the World

Genetically modified (GM) crops have become a staple in modern agriculture, with farmers around the world planting genetically engineered varieties to address various agricultural challenges. This global tour explores the presence of GM crops on different continents.

North America

United States

The adoption of GM crops in the U.S. has been substantial since their introduction in the 1990s. Some of the most widely grown GM crops in the U.S. include:

- **Soybeans:** GM soybeans were among the first GM crops to be commercially planted. They are used for various purposes, including animal feed, food products, and industrial applications.

- **Maize (Corn):** GM maize, primarily engineered to resist pests and tolerate herbicides, is extensively grown in the U.S. It serves as a staple food ingredient, livestock feed, and a source of biofuels.

- **Cotton:** GM cotton is grown for its fibers and oil. It is engineered to resist certain insect pests.

- **Canola:** GM canola is used for oil production and is engineered for herbicide tolerance.

- **Sugar Beets:** GM sugar beets, engineered for herbicide resistance, are a source of sugar production.

- **Alfalfa:** GM alfalfa is grown as livestock feed and is engineered for herbicide resistance.

South America

Genetically modified (GM) crops have had a significant impact on agriculture in South America. Several countries in the region have become major producers of GM crops, particularly soybeans, maize (corn), cotton, and canola. Here's an overview of GM crops in South America:

1. Major GM Crops:

Soybeans, maize, cotton, and canola are the primary GM crops grown in South America. They are cultivated for various purposes, including food production, animal feed, and industrial applications. GM traits in these crops include resistance to pests and tolerance to specific herbicides.

2. Key Countries:

Several South American countries are significant producers of GM crops:

- **Brazil:** Brazil is one of the world's largest producers of GM crops, with a focus on soybeans, maize, and cotton. The country has experienced substantial growth in GM crop adoption, driven by increased yields and pest resistance.

- **Argentina:** Argentina is another major GM crop producer, primarily growing GM soybeans and maize. The adoption of GM crops has been instrumental in increasing agricultural productivity.

- **Paraguay:** Paraguay also produces GM soybeans, maize, and cotton, and GM crops play a vital role in the country's agricultural sector.

- **Uruguay:** Uruguay has seen the adoption of GM soybeans and maize, which has contributed to the growth of its agriculture sector.

- **Bolivia:** Bolivia cultivates GM soybeans and maize, though the adoption of GM crops has been a subject of debate and regulatory changes.

Brazil

Genetically modified (GM) crops have had a substantial impact on agriculture in Brazil. The country has become one of the world's largest producers of GM crops, particularly soybeans, maize (corn), and cotton. The adoption of GM crops in Brazil has brought both benefits and challenges. Here's an overview of GM crops in Brazil:

Major GM Crops:

- **Soybeans:** GM soybeans are one of the most significant GM crops in Brazil. They are primarily used for oil production, animal feed, and various industrial applications.

- **Maize (Corn):** GM maize is widely grown in Brazil. It is used for food products, livestock feed, and the production of biofuels.

- **Cotton:** GM cotton, engineered to resist certain insect pests, is a major crop in Brazil, contributing to the textile and agricultural sectors.

Key Features of GM Crop Adoption in Brazil:

- **Rapid Growth:** Brazil has experienced rapid growth in the adoption of GM crops over the years. This growth has been driven by increased yields, pest resistance, and the economic benefits associated with GM agriculture.

- **Export Focus:** The country is a major exporter of GM soybeans, which are crucial for both domestic use and international trade. Brazil plays a significant role in global soybean production.

- **Diverse Agriculture:** Brazil's vast and diverse climate and geography allow for the cultivation of various GM crops across different regions of the country.

Argentina:

Genetically modified (GM) crops have played a pivotal role in Argentina's agricultural landscape. It has embraced GM technology, primarily in soybeans, maize (corn), and cotton. Here's an overview of

GM crops in Argentina:

1. Major GM Crops:

- **Soybeans:** GM soybeans are the most extensively cultivated GM crop in Argentina. These soybeans are primarily used for oil production, animal feed, and industrial applications.

- **Maize (Corn):** GM maize is also widely grown in Argentina. It is used for various purposes, including livestock feed, food products, and biofuels.

- **Cotton:** GM cotton, engineered for insect resistance, is an important crop in Argentina's textile and agricultural sectors.

2. Key Features of GM Crop Adoption in Argentina:

- **Rapid Adoption:** Argentina has experienced rapid and widespread adoption of GM crops, with the technology being embraced by both large and small-scale farmers.

- **Export-Oriented Agriculture:** Argentina is a significant exporter of GM soybeans, particularly to international markets like China and Europe. This has a substantial impact on the country's economy.

Europe

Spain

Spain is one of the European countries that has been cultivating genetically modified (GM) crops, although the cultivation of GM crops is significantly more limited in Europe compared to other parts of the world. Here is an overview of GM crops in Spain:

1. GM Crops Cultivated in Spain:

Spain has primarily focused on the cultivation of GM maize (corn) and GM cotton. These crops have been genetically modified to resist certain pests, primarily the European corn borer in the case of GM maize. Spain also conducts field trials of other GM crops for research purposes.

Key Features of GM Crop Adoption in Spain:

- **Limited Cultivation:** GM crop cultivation in Spain has been limited compared to countries like the United States and Argentina. Cultivation is primarily concentrated in certain regions of the country.

- **Research and Field Trials:** Spain has been active in conducting research and field trials for GM crops. This research aims to assess the performance and potential benefits of GM crops under local conditions.

- **Challenges and Opposition:** The cultivation of GM crops in Spain has faced challenges and opposition from various environmental and anti-GMO groups, as well as some regions and municipalities declaring themselves GMO-free zones.

Asia

India

Genetically modified (GM) crops have been a topic of discussion and research in India, and their cultivation has seen both acceptance and challenges. Here's an overview of the situation regarding GM crops in India:

GM Crops in India: India has primarily focused on the cultivation of GM cotton, with the introduction of Bt cotton being a significant milestone. Bt cotton is genetically modified to produce a protein toxic to certain insect pests, providing resistance to bollworms.

Adoption of Bt Cotton: The adoption of Bt cotton in India has been extensive, with millions of farmers planting this GM crop. Bt cotton has shown positive impacts, such as increased cotton yields and a reduction in the use of chemical pesticides.

China

China has been actively involved in the research and cultivation of genetically modified (GM) crops. The country has a significant stake in the global GM crop landscape, with both GM cotton and GM food crops being produced. Here's an overview of the situation regarding GM crops in China:

GM Crops in China: China has primarily focused on the cultivation of GM cotton, but it has also conducted research and field trials on GM food crops, such as rice, maize (corn), and soybeans.

Adoption of GM Cotton: GM cotton has been widely adopted in China. The primary GM cotton variety cultivated is Bt cotton, which is genetically modified to produce a protein toxic to certain insect pests, providing resistance to bollworms. Bt cotton has demonstrated positive impacts, such as increased cotton yields and a reduction in the use of chemical pesticides.

Philippines

The Philippines has been actively involved in the research and cultivation of genetically modified (GM) crops. The country has adopted several GM crops, particularly GM maize (corn) and GM eggplant. Here's an overview of the situation regarding GM crops in the Philippines:

GM Crops in the Philippines: The Philippines has primarily focused on the cultivation of GM maize and GM eggplant. These crops have been genetically modified to provide resistance to specific pests.

Adoption of GM Maize: GM maize, specifically Bt maize, has been widely adopted in the Philippines. Bt maize is engineered to produce a protein toxic to certain insect pests, providing resistance to corn borers and other pests. The adoption of Bt maize has resulted in increased yields and a reduction in the use of chemical pesticides.

Adoption of GM Eggplant: GM eggplant, known as Bt talong or Bt brinjal, has also been approved for commercial cultivation in the Philippines. It is engineered to resist the eggplant fruit and shoot borer, a significant pest in eggplant farming.

Research and Field Trials: The Philippines has conducted research and field trials for various GM crops, including rice, papaya, and sugarcane. These trials aim to assess the performance, safety, and potential benefits of GM crops under local conditions.

Africa

South Africa

South Africa has been actively involved in the cultivation of genetically modified (GM) crops for several years. The adoption of GM crops in the country has had significant impacts on agriculture, offering both benefits and challenges. Here's an overview of the situation regarding GM crops in South Africa:

Major GM Crops: South Africa primarily cultivates GM maize (corn), GM soybeans, and GM cotton. These crops are genetically modified for various traits, such as resistance to specific pests and tolerance to herbicides.

Adoption of GM Crops: The adoption of GM crops in South Africa has been substantial, with GM maize and GM soybeans being widely grown. GM cotton is also cultivated but to a lesser extent. The adoption of GM crops has demonstrated several benefits, including increased yields and reduced pest damage.

Nigeria

Nigeria, like many other countries, has been exploring the potential of genetically modified (GM) crops as a means to improve agricultural productivity and food security. While the adoption of GM crops in Nigeria is still relatively limited compared to some other countries, there has been ongoing research and development in this field. Here is an overview of the situation regarding GM crops in Nigeria:

GM Crops in Nigeria: Nigeria has primarily focused on the development and field trials of GM crops. Various GM crop research projects have been initiated to address specific agricultural challenges and increase crop yields.

Adoption of GM Crops: Commercial cultivation of GM crops in Nigeria is relatively limited. Field trials have been conducted for various GM crops, including GM cowpea (African black-eyed pea), GM cassava, and GM sorghum, among others. These crops are developed with traits such as resistance to pests and diseases.

Australia

Australia

Australia has been involved in the research and commercial cultivation of genetically modified (GM) crops, particularly GM cotton and GM canola. Here's an overview of the situation regarding GM crops in Australia:

GM Crops in Australia: Australia has primarily focused on the commercial cultivation of GM cotton and GM canola. These crops have been genetically modified to possess traits such as insect resistance, herbicide tolerance, and improved yield.

Adoption of GM Crops:

- **GM Cotton:** GM cotton, specifically Bt cotton, has been widely adopted in Australia. Bt cotton is engineered to produce a protein toxic to certain insect pests, providing resistance to cotton bollworms. The adoption of Bt cotton has demonstrated several benefits, including increased cotton yields and a reduction in the use of chemical pesticides.

- **GM Canola:** GM canola, engineered for herbicide tolerance, is also cultivated in Australia. This technology simplifies weed management and provides economic benefits to farmers.

The Impact on Nutrition Worldwide

The impact of GM crops on nutrition varies depending on the crop and region. In many developed and developing countries, GM crops have improved agricultural productivity and food security by reducing losses from pests and diseases. Biofortified GM crops, like Golden Rice and Bt cowpea, have the potential to address specific nutritional deficiencies, particularly in regions with limited access to diverse diets.

However, concerns about the nutritional quality of GM foods, labeling, and long-term health effects persist in some regions. The presence of GM ingredients in processed foods also raises questions about transparency and consumer choice.

GM crops are a global phenomenon, with different regions adopting them to address specific agricultural and nutritional challenges. While they have the potential to improve nutrition and food security, responsible regulation and public awareness are crucial to ensure that the benefits of GM crops are realized while addressing valid concerns about health, the environment, and food transparency.

Chapter 5

Unraveling the Label Mystery

The labeling of genetically modified (GM) or genetically engineered (GE) foods varies significantly around the world, reflecting the diverse regulatory approaches, public attitudes, and trade considerations of different countries and regions. Here is an overview of the current state of GM food labeling across the world:

European Union (EU)

Genetically modified (GM) food labeling in the European Union (EU) is one of the most stringent and comprehensive labeling systems in the world. The EU has established a robust regulatory framework for GM food labeling to ensure transparency and provide consumers with the information they need to make informed choices. Here is an overview of GM food labeling in the EU:

Mandatory Labeling: In the EU, GM food labeling is mandatory, and all food and feed products containing or consisting of genetically modified organisms (GMOs) or derived from GMOs must be labeled. This includes both processed and unprocessed foods, as well as animal feed. Mandatory labeling extends to all GM ingredients present in the final product, regardless of their quantity.

Labeling Threshold: The EU has set a specific threshold for GM content, and products must be labeled if they contain more than 0.9% of approved GM ingredients. This threshold is known as the "adventitious or technically unavoidable presence of GM material." If a product contains less than this threshold, labeling is not required. However, it's important to note that any detectable presence of unauthorized GM material, even at levels below 0.9%, is not allowed in the EU.

Labeling Requirements: GM food labels in the EU must contain specific information, including:

a. A statement that the food or feed contains GMOs.

b. The name of the GMO.

c. Any allergen information (if applicable).

d. Specific labeling rules for GM enzymes used in food processing.

Tracing and Identification: The EU requires a robust system for tracing and identifying GMOs at all stages of production and distribution. This ensures that all GM products can be tracked back to their origin and that any authorized GMOs can be accurately labeled.

Penalties for Non-Compliance:

EU member states are responsible for enforcing GM food labeling regulations. Non-compliance with labeling requirements can result in penalties, including fines or product recalls.

Public and Consumer Involvement: The EU values public and consumer involvement in decision-making processes related to GM foods. The public is encouraged to participate in consultations and express their views on issues related to GM food safety and labeling.

Precautionary Principle:

The EU follows the precautionary principle when it comes to GM crops and foods. If there is scientific uncertainty regarding the safety of a GM product, it may be subject to further evaluation and stringent safety assessments before being approved for cultivation or import.

Regulation of Novel Foods: Novel foods, including GM foods, are subject to a separate EU regulation that requires a safety assessment and authorization before they can be placed on the market. This regulation includes labeling requirements for novel foods.

Certification and Inspection: The EU establishes certification and inspection procedures to ensure that GM foods meet the necessary safety and labeling standards before entering the market.

European Union GMO Identifiers

In the European Union (EU), genetically modified organisms (GMOs) are identified and tracked using several key identifiers and information, including:

1. **Unique Identifier (EU GMID):** The Unique Identifier, also known as the EU GMID (European Union Genetically Modified Organism Identifier), is a primary identifier for GMOs in the EU. It includes the following components:

- **"E" followed by a Four-Digit Number:** The "E" stands for "European," and the four-digit number uniquely identifies the GMO.

- **"MY":** These letters stand for "Modification Year" and indicate the year when the GMO was first authorized.

- **Another Four-Digit Number:** This number distinguishes between different authorizations for the same GMO in a given year.

2.   **Authorization Number:** Each GMO that receives approval for commercial use in the EU is assigned an authorization number. This number is issued by the European Commission, and it is unique to each authorized GMO.

3.   **GM Plant Register Number:** For genetically modified plants, a register number is assigned in accordance with the EU's GM Plant Register. This number is used to identify individual GM plant varieties.

4.   **Event Codes:** GMOs can also be identified by event codes. Event codes are specific alphanumeric codes that represent the unique transformation events from which GMOs are derived.

Each transformation event corresponds to a specific genetic modification.

GM food labeling in the European Union is based on the principles of transparency, safety, and consumer choice. The EU's strict regulations require clear and accurate labeling of all GM food and feed products, with specific labeling requirements for the identification of GMOs. These regulations are designed to provide consumers with the information they need to make informed choices while ensuring the safety and traceability of GM products in the European market.

Australia and New Zealand

Genetically modified (GM) food labeling in Australia and New Zealand is governed by the Australia New Zealand Food Standards Code. This regulatory framework aims to ensure that consumers have access to clear and accurate information about the presence of GM ingredients in the food they purchase. Here is an overview of GM food labeling in Australia and New Zealand:

Mandatory GM Food Labeling: In Australia and New Zealand, GM food labeling is mandatory. Food products that contain GM ingredients must be labeled to provide consumers with information about their presence.

Labeling Threshold: There is a specific threshold for GM labeling in these countries. Products must be labeled if they contain novel DNA or novel protein resulting from genetic modification. This includes both direct modifications and unintended changes. The threshold for mandatory labeling is the presence of 1% or more of GM material.

Labeling Requirements: The labeling requirements for GM foods in Australia and New Zealand are comprehensive and include the following elements:

1. The word "genetically modified" or "genetically engineered" must be prominently displayed on the label, indicating the presence of GM

ingredients.

2. A statement about the presence of GM ingredients must be included, such as "contains genetically modified [name of the organism]."

3. Clear identification of the specific GM organism used in the product, such as "genetically modified soy."

4. Allergen labeling if applicable. If a GM food contains allergenic proteins or substances, this information must be clearly indicated on the label.

5. Labeling requirements extend to all foods, including processed and unprocessed products, as well as animal feed.

Exemptions: There are certain exemptions to the GM labeling requirements in Australia and New Zealand. These include:

- **Highly refined products:** Highly processed or refined products where GM DNA or protein is no longer detectable are exempt from labeling.

- **Incidental presence:** Products with an incidental presence of GM material, which is unintentional and below the 1% threshold, are exempt.

- **Organic foods:** Certified organic products that comply with organic standards may be exempt from labeling if they meet specific criteria.

Public Consultation and Involvement: The process for establishing and amending GM food labeling standards in Australia and New Zealand includes public consultation and stakeholder input. This ensures that the views and concerns of the public and industry are taken into account when developing or revising regulations.

Enforcement and Penalties: Enforcement of GM food labeling regulations is the responsibility of food regulatory agencies in both countries. Non-compliance can lead to penalties, including fines and product recalls.

Coordinated Approach: Australia and New Zealand maintain a coordinated approach to GM food labeling through their joint food standards agency, Food Standards Australia New Zealand (FSANZ). FSANZ plays a central role in the development and implementation of labeling standards for GM foods.

GM food labeling in Australia and New Zealand is characterized by clear, mandatory requirements that provide consumers with information about the presence of GM ingredients in their food. These regulations aim to balance consumer transparency with the need for practical labeling rules. Public consultation and ongoing monitoring of developments in biotechnology and genetic modification contribute to the effectiveness of the GM food labeling system in these countries.

Brazil

Genetically modified (GM) food labeling in Brazil reflects the country's approach to regulation and transparency in the context of GM crops and food products. Brazil is a major producer of GM crops, particularly soybeans, maize, and cotton, and its approach to GM food labeling has evolved over time. Here is an overview of GM food labeling in Brazil:

Mandatory Labeling for GM Foods: In Brazil, GM food labeling is mandatory. This means that food products containing GM ingredients or derivatives of GM crops must be labeled to inform consumers of their presence.

Labeling Threshold: Brazil has a specific threshold for GM labeling. Products must be labeled if they contain 1% or more of GM material. This threshold is similar to that of some other countries, including Australia and New Zealand.

Labeling Requirements: The labeling requirements for GM foods in Brazil include:

1. **Specific Statement:** The label must include a statement indicating that the product contains genetically modified ingredients. Common wording includes "contém transgênicos" (contains transgenics) or "produto produzido a partir de soja transgênica" (product produced from transgenic soy).

2. **Clear Identification:** The label should clearly identify the specific GM ingredient used in the product, such as "genetically modified soy" or "transgenic maize."

3. **Allergen Labeling:** If a GM food contains allergenic proteins or substances, this information must be clearly indicated on the label to ensure consumer safety.

4. **Processed and Unprocessed Foods:** GM labeling requirements apply to both processed and unprocessed foods, ensuring that consumers receive information about GM ingredients in all types of products.

Exemptions: Brazilian regulations provide some exemptions from GM food labeling:

- Highly processed or refined products

where GM DNA or protein is no longer detectable are exempt from labeling.

- Products with an incidental presence of GM material that is unintentional and falls below the 1% threshold are exempt.

- Animal products from animals fed with GM feed are generally exempt from labeling, as long as the final product does not contain GM material above the threshold.

Enforcement and Penalties: Enforcement of GM food labeling regulations in Brazil is overseen by regulatory agencies such as the Brazilian Ministry of Agriculture, Livestock, and Food Supply (MAPA) and the National Health Surveillance Agency (ANVISA). Non-compliance with labeling regulations can result in penalties, including fines and product recalls.

Public Awareness and Education: In Brazil, as in many other countries, there is an ongoing effort to educate the public about GM foods and labeling. Consumer awareness and understanding of GM labeling are important aspects of ensuring the effectiveness of the regulatory framework.

Coexistence and Traceability: The coexistence of GM and non-GM agriculture is an important consideration in Brazil. The country has developed guidelines to minimize the unintended mixing of GM and non-GM crops and to ensure traceability throughout the supply chain.

GM food labeling in Brazil is characterized by mandatory requirements that aim to provide consumers with information about the presence of GM ingredients in their food. These regulations have evolved to accommodate Brazil's significant role in global GM crop production while ensuring transparency and consumer choice. Public awareness, enforcement, and ongoing monitoring are essential aspects of the

Brazilian approach to GM food labeling.

China

Genetically modified (GM) food labeling in China is subject to government regulations and plays a crucial role in ensuring transparency and consumer choice. China is a significant producer and consumer of GM crops, and its approach to GM food labeling reflects the government's commitment to food safety and public awareness. Here is an overview of GM food labeling in China:

Mandatory Labeling for GM Foods: In China, GM food labeling is mandatory. This means that any food product containing GM ingredients or derivatives must be labeled to inform consumers of their presence.

Labeling Threshold: China has a specific threshold for GM labeling. Products must be labeled if they contain 3% or more of GM ingredients. This threshold represents a less strict requirement than some other countries, such as Australia and New Zealand, which have a 1% threshold.

Labeling Requirements: The labeling requirements for GM foods in China include:

1. **Specific Statement:** The label must include a statement indicating that the product contains genetically modified ingredients. Common wording includes "转基因" (genetically modified) or "含有转基因成分" (contains genetically modified ingredients).

2. **Clear Identification:** The label should clearly identify the specific GM ingredient used in the product, such as "转基因大豆" (genetically modified soy) or "含有转基因玉米" (contains genetically modified maize).

3. **Allergen Labeling:** If a GM food contains allergenic proteins or substances, this information must be clearly indicated on the label to ensure consumer safety.

4. **Processed and Unprocessed Foods:** GM labeling requirements apply to both processed and unprocessed foods, ensuring that consumers receive information about GM ingredients in all types of products.

Enforcement and Penalties: The enforcement of GM food labeling regulations in China is overseen by government agencies, including the China National Center for Food Safety Risk Assessment (CFSA) and the State Administration for Market Regulation. Non-compliance with labeling regulations can result in penalties, including fines and product recalls.

Public Awareness and Education: China has made efforts to educate the public about GM foods and labeling. Consumer awareness and understanding of GM labeling are considered important for the effectiveness of the regulatory framework. Public awareness campaigns and educational initiatives are conducted to inform consumers about the benefits and safety of GM foods.

International Trade Considerations: China is a major importer of GM crops, such as soybeans and maize, for use in animal feed and food processing. Meeting labeling requirements is essential for both domestically produced and imported GM food products to be sold in the Chinese market. This ensures consistency with international trade standards and agreements.

GM food labeling in China is characterized by mandatory requirements designed to provide consumers with information about the presence of GM ingredients in their food. These regulations reflect China's significant role in both the production and consumption of GM crops. Public awareness, enforcement, and adherence to international trade standards are key aspects of the Chinese approach to GM food labeling, as the country continues to develop and adapt its regulations to meet evolving needs and consumer demands.

United States

Genetically modified (GM) food labeling in the United States has been a subject of discussion and regulatory development for many years. The U.S. approach to GM food labeling has evolved over time, balancing the need for transparency with the complexities of a diverse and extensive food supply chain. Here is an overview of GM food labeling in the United States:

The National Bioengineered Food Disclosure Standard:

In 2016, the U.S. Congress passed the National Bioengineered Food Disclosure Standard, which established federal regulations for GM food labeling. The law was signed by President Barack Obama and is also known as the GMO labeling law.

Mandatory Labeling:

The National Bioengineered Food Disclosure Standard mandates that some GM food products be labeled. However, the use of the term "genetically modified" or "GMO" is avoided in favor of "bioengineered" or

"BE." This labeling is required for foods that contain bioengineered genetic material and do not meet certain exceptions.

Labeling Threshold:

The threshold for labeling in the U.S. is the presence of bioengineered genetic material that is detectable. If a food product contains genetic material from a bioengineered organism, it may need to be labeled.

Labeling Requirements:

The specific requirements for GM food labeling in the U.S. include:

1. **Disclosure on Packaging:** Food manufacturers must disclose the presence of bioengineered ingredients on the product's packaging. This disclosure

can take the form of text, symbols, or electronic Quick Response (QR) codes that consumers can scan with a smartphone for more information.

2. **Clear Disclosure:** The labeling must provide clear information about the presence of bioengineered ingredients in the product.

Exemptions:

In the United States, the National Bioengineered Food Disclosure Standard (NBFDS) sets guidelines for labeling genetically modified (GM) or bioengineered foods. The NBFDS includes a threshold for the presence of bioengineered genetic material in food products. Foods with very low levels of bioengineered genetic material are exempted from GM food labels if they fall below this threshold. Here are some examples of such exempted food products:

1. **Processed Foods with Traces of GM Ingredients:** Many processed foods may contain minimal traces of GM ingredients, typically derived from common GM crops like corn, soy, canola, and sugar beets. These trace amounts are often below the threshold and do not require GM labeling. For instance, foods with small amounts of corn syrup or soy lecithin are often exempt.

2. **Highly Refined Ingredients:** Highly refined products that no longer contain detectable genetic material are exempt from GM labeling. An example is refined

soybean oil, which is processed to the extent that it lacks GM DNA or proteins.

3.   **Alcohol:** Alcoholic beverages, such as beer or spirits, that are derived from GM crops like corn (used for distillation) are generally exempt from GM labeling requirements, as the refining and processing removes most of the genetic material.

4.   **Food Additives:** Some food additives and processing aids, like enzymes or flavorings, may be derived from GM microorganisms. However, if these additives no longer contain detectable genetic material, they are exempt from GM labeling.

It's important to note that the specific regulations regarding GM food labeling may evolve, and the exempted categories can vary. Consumers who are concerned about GM ingredients in their food should review product labels or seek out products with non-GMO or organic certification if they want to avoid bioengineered genetic material entirely. Additionally, these regulations are subject to change, so it's advisable to stay informed about the latest developments in GM food labeling standards and regulations.

Voluntary Labeling: Food manufacturers may voluntarily label their products as "non-GMO" or "GMO-free" if their products meet specific criteria and adhere to labeling guidelines established by non-governmental organizations.

Enforcement and Penalties: The enforcement of GM food labeling regulations in the U.S. is overseen by the U.S. Department of Agriculture (USDA). Non-compliance with labeling regulations can result in penalties, including fines.

State-Specific Regulations: Before the federal labeling law was passed, some U.S. states had introduced their own GM food labeling requirements. However, the federal law supersedes these state laws to create uniformity in labeling standards across the country.

GM food labeling in the United States is characterized by the National

Bioengineered Food Disclosure Standard, which established federal regulations for labeling bioengineered foods. This law balances the need for transparency with the diverse nature of the U.S. food supply chain. It provides consumers with information about the presence of bioengineered ingredients in their food, allowing them to make informed choices while avoiding overly burdensome labeling requirements for the food industry.

Canada

Canada has a system of voluntary labeling for genetically modified (GM) foods, which means that GM food labeling is not mandatory. However, there are certain regulations and guidelines in place to govern the labeling of GM foods in Canada. Here's a detailed discussion of GM food labeling in Canada:

1. Voluntary Labeling:

- Canada does not require mandatory labeling of GM foods that have been assessed and approved as safe for consumption. This means that, in most cases, GM foods do not need to be labeled as such.

- The Canadian government's stance is that mandatory labeling is only necessary when there is a clear health or safety concern, or when the nutritional composition of the GM food differs significantly from its conventional counterpart.

- The decision to label a GM food product is typically left to the discretion of the manufacturer, distributor, or retailer. They may choose to label a product as containing GM ingredients or as "GMO" or "genetically modified."

2. Allergen Labeling:

- Canadian food labeling regulations require manufacturers to disclose the presence of common allergens, such as soy, wheat, peanuts, tree nuts, milk, eggs, fish, and shellfish. This is intended to protect consumers with food allergies.

- If a GM food product contains an allergenic GM ingredient (e.g., GM soy), it may be labeled to indicate the presence of the allergen, but it may not be specifically labeled as GM.

3. Non-GMO Labeling:

- Some manufacturers and producers in Canada choose to label their products as "Non-GMO" or "GMO-free" to cater to consumers who prefer non-genetically modified foods. This is a voluntary initiative and is not required by law.

- Non-GMO labeling is not regulated as strictly as mandatory allergen labeling, and the criteria for such labels may vary among products and companies. Certification by non-GMO verification organizations is one way to provide assurance to consumers.

4. Organic Labeling:

- Organic foods in Canada, certified by organizations like the Canada Organic Regime, are, by default, non-GMO. The organic standards typically prohibit the use of genetically modified ingredients.

- Products labeled as "organic" must meet specific organic standards, including restrictions on the use of GM ingredients.

5. Future Developments:

- The landscape of GM food labeling in Canada may evolve over time in response to public demand, scientific developments, and international trade considerations.

- Regulatory agencies like the Canadian Food Inspection Agency (CFIA) and Health Canada continue to monitor and assess the safety of GM foods and may adapt regulations accordingly.

It's important to note that the absence of mandatory GM labeling does not imply that GM foods are unsafe. Health Canada conducts safety assessments for GM foods to ensure their safety for human consumption. Additionally, labeling regulations and guidelines may have evolved since my last update, so it's advisable to consult the most current sources or relevant regulatory agencies for the latest information on GM food labeling in Canada.

India

India has specific regulations for the labeling of genetically modified (GM) foods. The labeling of GM foods in India is mandatory, and it is regulated by the Food Safety and Standards Authority of India (FSSAI). Here's a discussion of GM food labeling in India:

1. Mandatory GM Food Labeling:

- In India, it is mandatory to label all food products that contain genetically modified organisms (GMOs) or GM ingredients. This includes both packaged and non-packaged food products.

- The GM food labeling regulations are in place to ensure that consumers are informed about the presence of GM ingredients in the food they purchase.

2. Labeling Requirements:

- GM food labels in India must contain specific information, including the words "genetically modified" or "GM" on the label. The label must clearly indicate that the product contains GM ingredients.

- Additionally, the label must provide information about the GM content as a percentage of the total ingredients in the food product.

- If a food product contains multiple GM ingredients, each GM ingredient must be individually labeled with the percentage of GM content.

3. Threshold for Labeling:

- India has established a threshold for labeling GM foods. If a food product contains GM ingredients in an amount equal to or exceeding 5% of the total ingredients, it must be labeled as a GM food.

4. Non-Packaged Foods:

- The labeling requirements apply not only to packaged foods but also to non-packaged or loose foods, such as fruits and vegetables. In the case of non-packaged foods, information about GM content must be provided to consumers at the point of purchase.

5. Exemptions:

- Some products are exempt from GM labeling requirements in India, including animal products derived from animals fed with GM feed, as long as the GM material cannot be detected in the final product.

6. Enforcement:

- The FSSAI is responsible for enforcing GM food labeling regulations in India. Food manufacturers and distributors are required to comply with these regulations, and non-compliance can result in penalties.

7. Public Awareness:

- The FSSAI and other organizations in India work to raise public awareness about GM foods and their labeling requirements. This includes educating consumers about how to read and interpret GM food labels.

It's essential to note that regulations and policies can change over time. Therefore, for the most current and detailed information regarding GM food labeling in India, it is advisable to refer to the official website of the Food Safety and Standards Authority of India (FSSAI) or consult with relevant government authorities.

Argentina: Argentina has limited GM food labeling, and it primarily focuses on allergenic ingredients. It has faced criticism for not having stricter labeling requirements.

Japan: Japan has labeling requirements for GM foods but has relatively higher thresholds for labeling than the EU. Some GM foods are exempt from labeling, depending on their genetic makeup.

South Korea: South Korea has labeling requirements for GM foods, but they apply to certain products only, such as highly processed foods.

Russia: Russia has voluntary labeling for GM foods but has not enforced strict regulations on GM labeling.

African Countries: Many African countries have limited or no GM food labeling regulations. However, there is increasing interest in adopting labeling requirements and strengthening regulatory frameworks.

Several Other Countries: Many countries have limited or no GM food labeling, often due to regulatory and infrastructure limitations or the absence of public consensus on the issue.

It's important to note that the state of GM food labeling continues to evolve. Some countries are considering or implementing changes to their labeling regulations to enhance transparency and meet consumer demands for more information about the presence of GM ingredients in their food. Additionally, international trade agreements and harmonization efforts play a role in shaping labeling requirements and global trade of GM foods. As public awareness and concerns about GM foods grow, labeling will likely remain a subject of ongoing debate and adaptation in countries around the world.

Chapter 6

Nutritional Changes in GM Foods

Genetic modification has the potential to influence the nutritional content of foods in various ways. While the primary aim of genetic modification is often to enhance traits like pest resistance or yield, the resulting changes can have a direct or indirect impact on the nutritional quality of these foods. In this chapter, we will explore the specifics of how genetic modification can influence the nutritional content of our favorite foods.

Increased Nutrient Levels

One of the notable goals of genetic modification is to enhance the nutritional value of crops. This is achieved through the introduction or overexpression of genes responsible for the synthesis of specific nutrients. Some key examples include:

- **Golden Rice**: Engineered to contain higher levels of beta-carotene, a precursor of vitamin A. This is especially important in regions where vitamin A deficiency is prevalent.

- **Biofortified Crops**: Genetic engineering has been employed to enhance the nutritional content of crops, including iron-fortified beans and zinc-fortified rice. These modifications aim to address nutrient deficiencies.

2. Reduced Anti-Nutrients

Some crops naturally contain compounds that can reduce the bioavailability of essential nutrients. Genetic modification can be used to reduce or eliminate these anti-nutrients, making it easier for the body to absorb essential nutrients. For example:

- **Low-Phytate Crops**: Phytic acid is an anti-nutrient that can hinder the absorption of minerals like iron and zinc. Genetic engineering has been used to develop crops with lower phytate levels, improving mineral bioavailability.

3. Enhanced Protein Quality

Genetic modification can improve the protein content and quality of crops. This is significant for those who rely on plant-based sources of protein. Specific examples include:

- **Soybeans with Balanced Amino Acids:** Researchers have developed soybean varieties with a more balanced amino acid profile, making them nutritionally superior.

4.Healthier Fats

Genetic modification can also influence the fatty acid composition of crops. For example, canola oil derived from genetically modified canola plants can have a lower saturated fat content, making it a healthier choice.

5. Enhanced Shelf Life

While not directly related to nutritional content, genetic modification can indirectly impact nutrition by increasing the shelf life of foods. By reducing spoilage and waste, it ensures that nutritious foods remain available for longer periods.

6. Reduced Allergens

In some cases, genetic modification can help reduce allergenic proteins in crops, making these foods safer for those with allergies. This is particularly important for staple crops like wheat.

Genetic modification can significantly influence the nutritional content of our favorite foods. From enhanced nutrient levels and reduced anti-nutrients to healthier fats and balanced amino acids, genetic engineering has the potential to address nutrient deficiencies and improve the overall quality of the global food supply. However, the safety and regulatory aspects of these changes must be closely monitored to ensure that GM foods provide the intended nutritional benefits without introducing unintended consequences.

Chapter 7

The Human Health Connection

The introduction of genetically engineered (GE) or genetically modified (GM) foods has ignited a global conversation about the potential impact of these crops on human health. While genetically modified organisms (GMOs) offer numerous advantages in terms of increased crop yields and pest resistance, questions persist about their safety, particularly in relation to human consumption. Let's delves into the human health connection of GM foods, exploring the potential effects on allergies, toxins, and more.

The Allergy Question

The potential allergenicity of genetically modified (GM) foods is an important safety concern that has been a subject of rigorous evaluation and discussion within the field of biotechnology and food safety. Here is an overview of the allergy-related questions and considerations surrounding GM foods:

1. Introduction of Allergens:

- **Concern:** Genetic modification can introduce new proteins into a food crop. If one of these newly introduced proteins is an allergen (a substance that can trigger allergic reactions in susceptible individuals), it could pose a health risk.

- **Mitigation**: To address this concern, regulatory authorities in many countries, including the United States and the European Union, have established guidelines for assessing the potential allergenicity of GM foods. These guidelines require developers to compare the newly introduced proteins to a database of known allergens. If a GM food's newly introduced protein is substantially similar to a known allergen, it may undergo further evaluation or testing.

2. Cross-Allergenicity:

- **Concern**: In some cases, the introduced gene in a GM crop may come from a source known to cause allergies, such as a nut or a shellfish. There is concern that the introduction of such a gene into a different food crop could cause cross-allergenicity in individuals who are allergic to the source of the gene.

- **Mitigation:** This concern is addressed through allergenicity assessments and additional testing, including protein structure analysis and animal testing, to evaluate the potential for cross-reactivity with known allergens.

3. Unexpected Allergic Reactions:

- **Concern:** There is always a possibility of unexpected allergic reactions to GM foods. Allergenicity testing may not identify every potential allergen, and individual responses to novel proteins can vary.

- **Mitigation**: Regulatory agencies require developers to conduct allergenicity testing, including in vitro and in vivo studies, to assess the potential for allergenic reactions. However, risk can never be completely eliminated, so post-market surveillance and reporting systems are in place to monitor any adverse reactions once GM foods are on the market.

4. Labeling and Consumer Awareness:

- **Concern**: Consumers with allergies need accurate information about the contents of food products. Labeling of GM foods and clear disclosure of their GM status is crucial for consumers to make informed choices.

- **Mitigation:** Many countries have labeling regulations in place for GM foods, which require the disclosure of their GM status. Labeling provides consumers with the information needed to make choices based on their individual dietary needs and potential allergens.

It's important to note that regulatory agencies, such as the U.S. Food and Drug Administration (FDA) and the European Food Safety Authority (EFSA), conduct thorough evaluations to ensure the safety of GM foods, with a particular focus on allergenicity. Developers of GM crops are required to submit data on the proteins introduced into the crop, and these data are assessed for potential allergenicity.

While concerns about allergenicity are valid, the safety evaluation process for GM foods is designed to minimize the risks associated with introducing potential allergens. The goal is to ensure that GM foods are as safe for consumers as their non-GM counterparts.

Toxins and Anti-Nutrients

Toxins and anti-nutrients in genetically modified (GM) foods are potential concerns that need to be addressed during the development and safety assessment of GM crops. It's important to note that while GM foods go through extensive safety evaluations, unintended effects can occur, including the generation of toxins and anti-nutrients. Here's an overview of these concerns:

1. Generation of Toxins:

a. **Unintended Toxins**: During the process of genetic modification, the insertion or manipulation of genes can lead to unintended consequences. These unintended effects may result in the production of toxic compounds in the GM crop. For example, the activation or suppression of certain genes can inadvertently lead to the synthesis of harmful substances.

b. **Allergenic Proteins**: One concern is the potential introduction of allergenic proteins from one organism into another during genetic modification. This can happen when a gene from an allergenic source is introduced into a non-allergenic crop. If the newly introduced protein is allergenic, it can pose a risk to individuals with allergies.

c. **Secondary Metabolites**: Some GM crops produce secondary metabolites, which are chemical compounds not directly related to the plant's growth and development. These compounds can be toxic if consumed. For instance, certain types of Bt (Bacillus thuringiensis) crops produce Bt proteins as insecticides, which are generally considered safe for humans but could potentially cause allergic reactions in some individuals.

2. Generation of Anti-Nutrients:

a. **Phytates:** Some GM crops may unintentionally have higher levels of phytates. Phytates are compounds that can bind to minerals like iron, calcium, and zinc in the digestive system, making them less available for absorption. Increased phytate levels can reduce the nutritional quality of the crop.

b. **Tannins:** In some cases, genetic modifications can lead to higher levels of tannins. Tannins can interfere with the absorption of minerals, particularly iron, and can also affect protein digestibility.

c. **Protease Inhibitors:** GM crops with unintended alterations in protein content may have elevated levels of protease inhibitors. These compounds can interfere with protein digestion in the human gastrointestinal tract.

Addressing Toxins and Anti-Nutrients in GM Foods:

To mitigate the risks associated with toxins and anti-nutrients in GM foods, rigorous safety assessments are conducted before GM crops are approved for commercial use. These assessments involve molecular analysis, animal feeding studies, and allergenicity testing. Regulators, such as the U.S. FDA, the European Food Safety Authority (EFSA), and other relevant agencies, review the data and determine whether the GM crop poses any safety concerns.

Furthermore, researchers aim to minimize unintended effects by using advanced molecular techniques, conducting thorough genetic analyses, and employing bioinformatics tools to predict potential unintended changes in GM crops.

It's important to emphasize that while concerns regarding toxins and anti-nutrients in GM foods are valid, regulatory agencies and scientists take these issues seriously and employ stringent safety evaluations to ensure that GM crops are safe for human consumption. However, continuous monitoring and research are essential as the technology evolves and new GM crops are developed.

Nutrient Changes

Genetic modification also offers the potential to enhance the nutrient content of food. For example, Golden Rice has been developed to contain higher levels of provitamin A (beta-carotene), addressing vitamin A deficiency in regions where rice is a dietary staple. This innovation has the potential to reduce the prevalence of vitamin A deficiency, which can lead to blindness and other health problems. While GM foods have the potential to positively impact human health by addressing nutritional deficiencies, they also raise questions about their long-term effects on health and safety.

Regulatory Oversight

To address the complex and multi-faceted human health concerns associated with GM foods, countries around the world have established regulatory frameworks. These frameworks require safety assessments and allergenicity testing, as well as long-term health and environmental impact assessments before GM foods can enter the market.

In the United States, for instance, the Food and Drug Administration (FDA) evaluates GM foods to ensure they are safe for human consumption. The World Health Organization (WHO) and the Food and Agriculture Organization (FAO) also play significant roles in establishing international guidelines for GM food safety.

The human health connection with genetically engineered foods is a multifaceted issue, encompassing concerns related to allergies, toxins, anti-nutrients, and nutrient changes. While GM foods offer the potential to address global nutritional deficiencies and reduce the need for chemical pesticides, safety and regulatory oversight are of paramount importance.

The debate around GM foods remains a dynamic and evolving conversation, with science, regulation, and public awareness continuing to shape the future of genetically engineered crops. Research, transparency, and adherence to rigorous safety assessments are essential in ensuring that

GM foods contribute positively to human health without compromising safety and well-being. The continued evaluation of GM crops will be critical in addressing these health-related questions and providing consumers with safe and nutritious food choices.

Chapter 8

Feeding the Future

As the global population continues to grow, so does the demand for food. To meet the nutritional needs of billions of people while addressing the challenges of climate change, limited arable land, and diminishing natural resources, genetic engineering plays a pivotal role in shaping the future of agriculture. In this exploration, we discover how genetic engineering is at the forefront of efforts to ensure food security and sustainability for generations to come.

1. Increased Crop Yields

Genetic engineering has the potential to significantly boost crop yields. By introducing traits that enhance resistance to pests and diseases, as well as tolerance to adverse environmental conditions like drought and salinity, genetically modified (GM) crops can produce more food on the same amount of land. This is crucial for feeding a growing global population.

2. Pest and Disease Resistance

One of the most impactful applications of genetic engineering is the development of crops that can resist pests and diseases. For example, Bt crops, which contain genes from the bacterium Bacillus thuringiensis, produce proteins toxic to certain insect pests. This reduces the need for chemical pesticides, making agriculture more environmentally friendly and financially sustainable.

3. Drought Tolerance

With climate change leading to more frequent and severe droughts, crops that can withstand water stress are essential for food security. Genetic engineering can help create varieties of key crops that are more drought-tolerant, ensuring reliable harvests even in arid regions.

4. Improved Nutritional Value

Genetic engineering is utilized to enhance the nutritional value of crops. "Golden Rice," for instance, is engineered to produce beta-carotene, a precursor to vitamin A. This can help combat vitamin A deficiency, which is a significant public health concern in many developing countries.

5. Reduced Environmental Impact

GM crops that require fewer chemical inputs, such as herbicides and pesticides, can lead to a reduction in the environmental impact of agriculture. By minimizing chemical usage, genetic engineering can contribute to improved soil health, reduced water contamination, and less harm to non-target organisms.

6. Sustainable Agriculture

Genetic engineering supports sustainable agriculture by promoting practices that reduce waste and conserve resources. By extending the shelf life of crops through modifications, it's possible to reduce post-harvest losses and ensure more food reaches consumers.

Genetic engineering is a powerful tool for addressing the pressing challenges of global food security and sustainability. By increasing crop yields, enhancing nutritional content, and reducing the environmental impact of agriculture, genetic engineering plays a pivotal role in feeding the future. Responsible innovation and close attention to ethical, regulatory, and consumer considerations are essential to harness the full potential of genetic engineering in this critical endeavor.

Chapter 9

Beyond the Plate

Genetic engineering, with its potential to reshape agriculture and food production, has far-reaching implications that extend well beyond what's on our plates. In this chapter, we'll delves into the broader impact of genetic engineering, touching on economic, environmental, and ethical considerations that influence the adoption and regulation of genetically modified organisms (GMOs).

Economic Considerations

1. **Farmers' Income**: Genetic engineering can affect farmers' income by increasing crop yields and reducing input costs, such as pesticides. It can also open up new markets and export opportunities, contributing to economic growth.

2. **Seed Costs**: The concentration of biotechnology companies in the seed industry has led to concerns about rising seed costs and corporate control. Some argue that this limits the choices available to farmers and can have economic consequences.

3. **Market Access**: Access to international markets can be influenced by a country's stance on GMOs. Some countries restrict

the import of GM products, potentially affecting the ability of farmers to sell their crops abroad.

4. **Economic Disparities**: The adoption of GM crops can sometimes exacerbate economic disparities between large commercial farms that benefit from genetic engineering and small-scale or subsistence farmers who may not have access to the technology.

Environmental Implications

1. **Reduced Pesticide Use:** One of the environmental benefits of genetic engineering is the potential to reduce pesticide use. This can lead to fewer chemical residues in the environment and

less harm to non-target organisms.

2. **Conservation and Biodiversity:** The impact of GM crops on local ecosystems and biodiversity is a subject of debate. Monoculture GM crops can affect local ecosystems by reducing biodiversity, while some GM crops are designed to promote conservation efforts.

3. **Herbicide-Resistant Weeds**: The overuse of herbicide-resistant GM crops can lead to the emergence of herbicide-resistant weeds, which can be a concern for farmers and the environment.

4. **Gene Flow:** The transfer of genetic material from GM crops to non-GM crops through cross-pollination can raise concerns about preserving the genetic

purity of traditional and organic varieties.

Ethical Concerns

1. **Ownership and Control**: Ethical concerns include the corporate control of seeds and genetic resources. The concentration of genetic engineering technology in the hands of a few major agrochemical companies can limit the choices available to farmers.

2. **Transparency**: The transparency and labeling of GM products are important ethical considerations. Some argue that consumers have a right to know whether the food they are purchasing contains GMOs.

3. **Societal Divisions**: Genetic engineering has the potential to create societal divisions based on access to genetic enhancements or the benefits of GM crops.

4. **Unintended Consequences**: Unintended ecological consequences and long-term health effects are ethical concerns that necessitate thorough evaluation and monitoring of GM crops.

Genetic engineering reaches far "beyond the plate," with implications that encompass economics, the environment, and ethics. While it holds the potential to address food security and sustainability, it also brings challenges related to corporate control, environmental impact, and ethical considerations. Responsible innovation, regulatory oversight, and public awareness are essential for ensuring that the broader implications of genetic engineering are carefully considered and balanced to benefit both agriculture and society as a whole.

Chapter 10

Making Informed Choices

In a world where genetically engineered (GE) foods are increasingly prevalent, making informed choices about your diet is crucial for your health, values, and the environment. This chapter provides tips and strategies to help you navigate the complex landscape of GE foods and make educated decisions that align with your preferences and priorities.

1. Understand Genetically Engineered (GE) Foods

The first step in making informed choices is to educate yourself about GE foods. Learn what genetic engineering is, how it's used in agriculture, and the various types of GE crops that are commonly found in the food supply.

2. Read Labels

Many countries require the labeling of GE foods. Check product labels for statements like "contains genetically modified organisms (GMOs)" or "GMO-free." This will help you identify whether a product contains GE ingredients.

3. Consider Your Values

Your values and priorities should guide your choices. If you're concerned about the environmental impact of GE crops, choose products that align with sustainable farming practices. If you are concerned about allergies, opt for GM foods that does not contain the allergic substance, non-GMO or organic options.

4. Stay Informed

Stay up to date with the latest developments in the field of genetic engineering, regulatory changes, and scientific research. Being informed empowers you to make decisions that reflect your current knowledge and understanding.

5 Advocate for Transparency

Advocate for clear labeling and transparency in the food industry. Support organizations and policies that promote accurate and accessible information about GE foods.

6. Engage in Dialogue

Engage in conversations with others who have diverse perspectives on GE foods. These discussions can help you refine your understanding and encourage responsible decision-making.

7. Assess the Benefits and Risks

Consider the potential benefits and risks of GE foods for your specific circumstances. Assess how they align with your health, dietary preferences, and values.

8. Consult Health Professionals

If you have specific health concerns related to GE foods or other dietary considerations, consult with a healthcare professional or a registered dietitian. They can provide personalized guidance.

9. **Balance Your Choices**

Remember that genetic engineering is just one factor to consider in your diet. Balance your choices with other important factors like nutrition, taste, and cultural or dietary preferences.

Making informed choices in an age of genetically engineered foods is possible by understanding the technology, reading labels, seeking alternative products, and aligning your choices with your values and priorities. By staying informed and advocating for transparency, you can make dietary decisions that reflect your individual needs and values.

Chapter 11

The Future of Food

The future of food is undoubtedly intertwined with genetic engineering, and as we look ahead, several key trends and developments are likely to shape our diets in the coming years:

1. Nutrient-Rich and Biofortified Foods

Genetic engineering will continue to play a pivotal role in addressing nutrient deficiencies on a global scale. Biofortified crops, such as Golden Rice, will be just the beginning. We can expect the development of a wide range of nutrient-rich foods that can help combat malnutrition and improve public health.

2. Climate-Resilient Crops

With climate change posing an increasing threat to agriculture, genetic engineering will be used to develop crops that can thrive in more challenging conditions. Drought-tolerant, heat-resistant, and flood-resistant crops will become essential in ensuring food security.

3. Reduced Environmental Impact

Genetic engineering will lead to the development of crops that require fewer chemical inputs, such as pesticides and fertilizers. This will help reduce the environmental impact of agriculture, minimizing water pollution and harm to non-target species.

4. Personalized Nutrition

Advancements in genetic engineering may pave the way for personalized nutrition. Individualized diets based on genetic factors could become more common, with food tailored to meet specific health needs and preferences. Picture a scene in a doctor's office where two patients are receiving recommendations. One patient is handed a prescription for rice enriched with iron, while the other is advised to incorporate rice fortified with vitamin B into their diet. Quite fascinating, isn't it?

5. Synthetic Biology and Alternative Protein Sources

The future will likely see the rise of synthetic biology in food production. Lab-grown meat, plant-based meat alternatives, and microbial fermentation techniques will become increasingly important for addressing sustainability concerns and reducing the environmental footprint of food production.

6. Ethical Considerations and Transparency

As genetic engineering continues to evolve, ethical considerations will come to the forefront. Ensuring transparency in labeling and regulation will be essential in addressing public concerns and promoting consumer trust.

7. Global Collaboration and Regulatory Frameworks

International collaboration on genetic engineering and the development of uniform regulatory frameworks will become more critical as the global food supply chain becomes increasingly interconnected. Countries will work together to address challenges related to trade, food safety, and environmental sustainability.

8. Coexistence of GM and Non-GM Crops

Managing the coexistence of genetically modified and non-GM crops will be a significant challenge. Striking a balance that allows both systems to coexist peacefully, without cross-contamination, will be essential.

9. Consumer Education and Engagement

Consumer education will become more important than ever as genetic engineering continues to shape the food landscape. The public will need to be informed about the benefits, risks, and ethical considerations of GM foods.

10. Precision and Control

Advancements in genetic editing technologies, such as CRISPR-Cas9, will provide scientists with greater precision and control in modifying crop genomes. This will open up new possibilities for developing crops with targeted traits.

The future of food will be marked by a continued reliance on genetic engineering to address some of the most pressing challenges in agriculture. From improving nutrition and increasing crop resilience to reducing the environmental impact of food production, genetic engineering will be at the forefront of innovation in the food industry. As these developments continue, careful consideration of the ethical, environmental, and regulatory aspects of genetic engineering will be essential to ensure that it benefits both humanity and the planet.

Chapter 13

Behind the Scenes: Biotech in Agriculture

The agriculture and biotech industries play a vital role in providing food for a growing global population. Behind the scenes, these sectors are characterized by innovation, challenges, and intricate practices. This chapter offers insights into the inner workings of biotechnology in agriculture, shedding light on the practices and challenges faced by these industries.

Biotechnology in Agriculture: A Game-Changer

Biotechnology in agriculture refers to the application of genetic engineering and molecular biology techniques to modify crops, making them more resistant to pests, diseases, and environmental stresses, as well as improving their nutritional content. It has had a profound impact on food production, helping meet the demand of a world with a population exceeding 7 billion.

Key Practices in Biotechnology in Agriculture

1. **Genetic Modification (GM):** Genetic engineering involves the insertion of specific genes into plant genomes to confer desirable traits, such as pest resistance or drought tolerance. This practice has led to the creation of genetically modified (GM) crops.

2. **Plant Breeding**: Traditional plant breeding, complemented by biotechnological tools, is used to develop new crop varieties with improved yield, taste, and resistance to diseases. This process can take years or even decades.

3. **Pest Management**: Integrated pest management (IPM) techniques are employed to reduce the need for chemical pesticides. This includes the use of natural predators and crop rotation.

4. **Sustainable Agriculture**: The agriculture industry is increasingly focusing on sustainability, promoting practices like no-till farming, precision agriculture, and reduced water usage.

Challenges Faced by the Industry

1. **Regulatory Hurdles**: One of the primary challenges in the biotech-agriculture industry is navigating a complex web of regulations. Different countries have varying stances on GM crops, leading to trade difficulties and increased costs.

2. **Public Perception and Opposition**: Biotechnology in agriculture faces public skepticism and opposition. Concerns about food safety, environmental impact, and corporate control of seeds have fueled a contentious debate.

3. **Biodiversity and Monoculture**: The widespread adoption of GM crops, particularly monoculture GM varieties, can impact biodiversity by reducing the

diversity of crops in certain areas. This can have ecological consequences.

4. **Coexistence and Gene Flow**: Coexistence of GM and non-GM crops is a significant challenge, as the genetic material can cross-pollinate. Ensuring that farmers have the choice to grow GM or non-GM crops without cross-contamination is complex.

5. **Environmental Concerns**: While biotechnology can reduce the need for chemical pesticides, the overreliance on certain GM crops, like herbicide-resistant varieties, has led to herbicide-resistant weed development.

Future Trends

1. **Precision Agriculture**: Precision agriculture, which involves the use of technology and data to optimize farming practices, will continue to grow. It allows farmers to reduce input costs and increase yields.

2. **Gene Editing**: Emerging gene editing techniques, such as CRISPR-Cas9, will enable more precise and targeted genetic modifications, reducing unintended side effects.

3. **Climate-Resilient Crops**: As climate change poses a significant challenge, biotechnology will be harnessed to develop crops that can thrive in changing environmental conditions.

4. **Biofortification**: Genetic engineering will be used to enhance the nutritional content of staple crops, addressing malnutrition and public health issues.

The agriculture and biotech industries are essential for feeding the world's population. The practices and challenges in these industries involve innovation, regulation, and a constant push for sustainability. Addressing public concerns, promoting transparency, and balancing the benefits of biotechnology with its challenges are key considerations for the future of agriculture and biotechnology.

Chapter 14

GM Foods and the Environment

Genetically modified (GM) foods have sparked discussions and debates concerning their environmental impact and sustainability. In this chapter we'll discuss the key issues surrounding GM foods and their consequences on the environment.

Environmental Impact of GM Foods

1. **Reduced Pesticide Use:** One of the potential environmental benefits of GM crops is the reduction in pesticide use. Crops engineered to resist pests, like Bt cotton and Bt corn, can lead to decreased chemical pesticide application, which

reduces the associated environmental contamination.

2. **Conservation Tillage**: Some GM crops, particularly herbicide-resistant varieties, can be used with conservation tillage practices. Reduced tilling helps prevent soil erosion and reduces carbon dioxide emissions.

3. **Enhanced Crop Yields**: GM crops engineered for increased yield can help reduce the pressure on expanding agricultural lands. This can contribute to habitat conservation and potentially reduce deforestation.

4. **Drought Tolerance**: GM crops designed to withstand drought conditions can thrive in arid regions, potentially reducing

the pressure on water resources.

5. **Biofortification**: GM crops can be engineered to be more nutritious, addressing nutritional deficiencies and related health issues.

Sustainability Issues and Concerns

1. **Biodiversity**: Monoculture planting of GM crops can reduce biodiversity in agricultural landscapes, potentially impacting ecosystems and wildlife.

2. **Herbicide-Resistant Weeds**: The overuse of herbicide-resistant GM crops has led to the emergence of herbicide-resistant weeds. This poses challenges for farmers and requires the use of additional, often more potent, herbicides.

3. **Gene Flow:** Cross-pollination between GM and non-GM crops can lead to gene flow, potentially affecting non-GM and organic crops. Managing coexistence is crucial to prevent unintentional mixing.

4. **Loss of Traditional Varieties:** The adoption of GM crops has sometimes led to a decline in traditional crop varieties, which can have cultural, nutritional, and genetic diversity implications.

5. **Environmental Uncertainty:** The long-term environmental consequences of GM crops are still not fully understood. The introduction of novel genes into ecosystems can have unpredictable effects.

Balancing Sustainability and Innovation

Balancing the sustainability of agriculture with the need for innovation is a central challenge in the GM food debate. Some strategies to address these issues include:

- **Crop Rotation**: To prevent herbicide-resistant weeds and maintain soil health, farmers can practice crop rotation and use different GM and non-GM crops.

- **Buffer Zones**: Establishing buffer zones between GM and non-GM fields can help reduce gene flow.

- **Precision Agriculture**: Implementing precision agriculture techniques can optimize resource use, reduce environmental impact, and increase yields.

- **Sustainable Farming Practices:** Combining GM technology with sustainable farming practices, such as conservation tillage and organic farming, can help mitigate environmental concerns.

- **Regulation and Oversight:** Rigorous regulatory oversight is essential to assess the environmental safety of GM crops and ensure that they are developed responsibly.

GM foods have both environmental benefits and sustainability challenges. Their potential to reduce pesticide use, enhance crop yields, and address nutritional deficiencies is significant. However, addressing concerns related to biodiversity, herbicide-resistant weeds, gene flow, and the long-term environmental impact is essential. Balancing the benefits of genetic engineering with its environmental challenges is key to ensuring the sustainability of our food supply.

Chapter 15

The Way Forward

Genetically engineered (GE) foods have the potential to offer numerous benefits, from increased crop yields to improved nutritional content. However, they also raise concerns about safety, the environment, and long-term consequences. The way forward involves finding a delicate balance between reaping the benefits and mitigating the risks associated with GE foods while ensuring their positive impact on nutrition. Here are potential paths to navigate this complex issue:

1. **Rigorous Regulatory Oversight**

Effective regulatory oversight is crucial for ensuring the safety and proper labeling of GE foods. Government agencies should continue to rigorously assess the safety of GM crops for both human consumption and the environment. Transparency in the approval process, including comprehensive risk assessments, is essential.

2. **Long-Term Environmental Monitoring**

Long-term environmental monitoring of GM crops should be a standard practice. This will help identify and address any unintended ecological consequences and enable scientists to understand the full impact of these crops on the environment.

3. **Educating the Public**

Increasing public awareness and understanding of genetic engineering is vital. Efforts should focus on informing consumers about the benefits and risks of GM foods to help them make informed choices based on their own values and concerns.

4. **Promoting Sustainable Farming Practices**

The integration of genetic engineering with sustainable farming practices can help mitigate the environmental impact of GM crops. Encouraging crop rotation, conservation tillage, and agroecological approaches can foster more sustainable agriculture.

5. Coexistence Measures

Creating coexistence guidelines and practices to prevent gene flow between GM and non-GM crops is essential. These measures can help organic and non-GM farmers maintain the integrity of their crops.

6. Diversifying Crop Varieties

Promoting crop diversity by preserving traditional and heirloom varieties can help address concerns about the loss of genetic diversity caused by GM monocultures.

7. Fostering Collaboration

Collaboration among governments, scientists, biotechnology companies, and farmers is essential. By working together, these stakeholders can develop solutions that balance the benefits and risks of GM crops.

8. Advancing Gene Editing Technologies

Continued advancements in gene editing technologies, such as CRISPR-Cas9, can enhance precision and reduce unintended consequences in genetic modifications. Research in this area should be encouraged.

9. Ethical Considerations

The ethical considerations surrounding GM foods, such as corporate control of seeds and equitable distribution of benefits, should be addressed through responsible business practices, fair intellectual property rights, and international agreements.

10. Consumer Choice and Labeling

Supporting clear and transparent labeling practices empowers consumers to make informed choices about the foods they purchase. Access to accurate information on GM content enables individuals to align their dietary choices with their values.

11. Global Cooperation

Given the interconnected nature of the global food supply chain, international cooperation is necessary to harmonize regulations, facilitate trade, and address transboundary concerns related to GM crops.

The path forward involves a multifaceted approach that balances the benefits and risks of genetically engineered foods while ensuring their positive impact on nutrition. Rigorous regulation, environmental monitoring, education, sustainable practices, and ethical considerations all play a role in achieving this balance. By fostering collaboration, transparency, and informed decision-making, we can harness the potential of genetic engineering to address food security, nutritional needs, and environmental sustainability.

Conclusion

As we reach the end of our journey through the captivating world of engineered foods, one thing becomes abundantly clear: our plates have not merely been altered; they have been revolutionized. "The Genetic Plate: Exploring the World of Engineered Foods" has unveiled a world of agricultural ingenuity, scientific breakthroughs, and culinary possibilities that are as remarkable as they are controversial.

From the inception of genetically modified (GM) crops to their cultivation in fields across the globe, we've witnessed the extraordinary feats of human intellect and the resilience of nature's wonders. The ability to engineer our foods has granted us the power to adapt to the unpredictable challenges of a changing climate and to address the profound issue of global food security.

However, our exploration has not been without its share of critical questions and ethical dilemmas. We've navigated the complex terrain of allergenicity, environmental impacts, and the transparency of labeling, acknowledging that with each scientific stride, we must tread cautiously and responsibly.

In the end, "The Genetic Plate" is an invitation to continue the conversation, a call to scrutinize the choices we make, and a reminder that innovation, tempered with wisdom, holds the key to a healthier, more sustainable future. The genetic plate before us is both an opportunity and a challenge, and it is a testament to the indomitable spirit of human curiosity and adaptability.

As the curtain falls on our journey, the stage is set for the next act in the story of engineered foods. The world is watching, debating, and innovating. Our plates, once blank canvases, are now a tapestry of science and artistry. The culinary landscape is ever-evolving, and the genetic plate is a reflection of our unceasing quest for nourishment, progress, and a deeper understanding of the world around us.

Let us continue to explore, to question, and to savor the flavors of discovery, for the genetic plate is as much about our past as it is about our future. It is, in essence, a story of our ever-evolving relationship with the most fundamental and fascinating aspect of our lives—our food.